The 21-Day Consciousness Cleanse

Also by Debbie Ford

THE DARK SIDE OF THE LIGHT CHASERS

SPIRITUAL DIVORCE

THE SECRET OF THE SHADOW

THE RIGHT QUESTIONS

THE BEST YEAR OF YOUR LIFE

WHY GOOD PEOPLE DO BAD THINGS

The
21-Day
Consciousness
Cleanse

*A Breakthrough Program for Connecting
with Your Soul's Deepest Purpose*

Debbie Ford

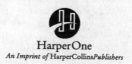

HarperOne
An Imprint of HarperCollinsPublishers

HarperOne

HarperCollins books may be purchased for educational, business, or sales promotional use. For information please write: Special Markets Department, HarperCollins Publishers, 10 East 53rd Street, New York, NY 10022.

HarperCollins website: http://www.harpercollins.com
HarperCollins®, ®, and HarperOne™ are
trademarks of HarperCollins Publishers

FIRST HARPERCOLLINS PAPERBACK EDITION PUBLISHED IN 2011
Designed by Level C

Library of Congress Cataloging-in-Publication Data
Ford, Debbie.
The 21-day consciousness cleanse : a breakthrough program for connecting with
your soul's deepest purpose / by Debbie Ford. — 1st ed.
p. cm.
ISBN 978–0–06–178369–2
1. Soul. 2. Self-actualization—Religious aspects. 3. Spiritual life. I. Title.
II. Title: Twenty-one-day consciousness cleanse.
BL290.F64 2009
158.1—dc22
2009012034

11 12 13 14 15 RRD (H) 10 9 8 7 6 5 4 3 2

This book was written to honor the writings and teachings
of Emmet Fox, a man whose wisdom, courage,
and strength gave me the wisdom, courage, and strength
to grow up, to let go, to let God, and to step into
my soul's passion. May his memory stay alive for
eternity and continue to turn the light on
for millions who still live in darkness.

Contents

Contents

The Future 177

The 21-Day Consciousness Cleanse

The 21-Day Consciousness Cleanse dedicates twenty-one days and nights to building a profound and intimate relationship with your soul and the infinite force that fuels you with the will to live your highest potential. It is a profound process for cleaning up the past, getting honest about the present, and envisioning a future unlike anything you've ever imagined. This process offers a full-immersion approach to spiritual renewal, emotional transformation, and reconnection with your deepest purpose. Designed to support you in letting go of all the false beliefs and assumptions that no longer serve you, this cleanse will guide you to a deep and profound relationship with the greatest love imaginable, a love that can occur only when you've made peace with yourself, others, and your life as it is right now. And I can tell you with unshakable confidence that it will work for you if you allow it to.

When you take the time to cleanse your physical body of accumulated stress and toxicity, you are rewarded with increased energy, vitality, and optimal functioning. In the same way, the Consciousness Cleanse is designed to purify your mind and emotions, bringing you enormous amounts of strength, confidence, and deep inner peace. Past hurts and resentments cloud your perception, while present-day distractions and ego-driven desires impede your ability to make good choices. The Consciousness Cleanse takes you on a journey of spiritual revitalization that will move your attention from the outside world back to your sacred interior. Like a physical cleanse, it will liberate you from the toxicity of the past, reconnect you with your soul's purpose, and gift you with the clarity and the inspiration to care for yourself like never before.

If you are ready to claim the gold that lies beneath the surface of the self that you know, you are in the perfect place. The most descriptive tale of this journey that I've ever encountered, one that comes fully to life, is a Buddhist story. In 1957, a monastery in Thailand was being relocated, and a group of monks was put in charge of moving a giant clay Buddha. In the midst of the move, one of the monks noticed a crack in its surface. Concerned about damaging the idol, the monks decided to wait a day before continuing with their task. One of the concerned monks came to further examine the giant statue. He shone his flashlight over the entire Buddha. When he reached the crack, he was astonished to see something reflected back at him. His curiosity aroused, the monk got a hammer and a chisel and began chipping away at the clay Buddha. As he knocked off piece after piece of clay, the Buddha got brighter and brighter. After hours of work, the monk looked up in amazement to see standing before him a huge solid-gold Buddha, a priceless treasure the likes of which had never been viewed before. Historians believe the Buddha had been covered with clay by Thai monks several hundred years earlier, before an attack by the Burmese army. The monks had covered the Buddha to protect it so it wouldn't get stolen. In the attack all the monks were killed, so it wasn't until this day that the real value of this great treasure was discovered.

Like the Buddha's clay covering, your outer shell serves to protect you from the world, while your real treasure, your soul's expression, is hidden within. Unknowingly, you hide your inner gold under a layer of human clay. And all you need to do to discover your real value—your soul's gold—is to have the courage to chip away at your outer shell, the persona of the human ego, piece by piece. The outer shell is what keeps you from seeing the real light that lies within—your purest essence, your power, and your real worth. Until you are able to see who and what you are at your core, you will settle for the self that you know, and may endure immense and often needless suffering.

Life will present you with countless opportunities to crack open to your divine nature. Most often, these appear during times of great distress. It is during these times that you have the opportunity to explore your inner world and begin the sacred process of becoming intimate with the totality of who you are, with your light as well as your darkness, your wins as well as your losses, your blessings as well as your disappointments. Your pain, when examined and embraced, becomes your spiritual director, inspiring new beginnings and ultimately leading you to emotional freedom and the liberation of your soul. But you don't have to wait until a moment of crisis or great pain to access the gift. There is another way to break through this often-impenetrable wall. The Consciousness Cleanse will help you to digest feelings and experiences you may have been running from for years. Each day of the cleanse is designed to call you into the vastness of who you are, unveiling the grandness and greatness of what is possible for your life. That is why it's imperative for you to unhook from the ego-driven life: so that you can reorganize your consciousness and live a soul-centered, heart-inspired life. And so I am asking you to unhook from the outer world and reconnect, on ever-deepening levels, with your inner world; to commit twenty-one days—*just twenty-one days of your entire life*—to your inner journey. It's such a small amount of time, but the payoffs are immeasurable. If you dare to clear the container to your consciousness, you will access feelings of love, compassion, joy, and deep peace. You will create the space for inspiration, creativity, and the genius of your soul to come through you. When your con-sciousness is clear, you can see that all you need to sustain and satisfy yourself already exists within—not on the outside of you, but on the inside of you.

If you are seriously considering the 21-Day Consciousness Cleanse, it is because, more than likely, you know there is far more for you than you are experiencing right now. Mediocrity in any area of your life is no longer an option, because either your pain is too great or your desire for having it all is too compelling. You want more, and you know you deserve more. You know there is something you're not getting, and you are ready to get it. So today is a perfect day for you to take back your power from the outer world, turn inward, and embark on the journey of reconnecting with the spirit that moves you. It is inside this structured program that you can clean out the container of your own consciousness, enabling you to experi-ence your most soulful self.

Love for the human journey—for all its challenges and joys—will chip away at the hardened shell of our limited self. I'll never forget hearing Waylon Jennings sing, "I was looking for love in all the wrong places." I was haunted for months by these words, because they triggered the recognition of a deeper truth—a truth that altered the very nature of my existence. I saw that he wasn't singing about just romantic love, but rather a universal truth that we all needed to come to terms with. Most of us *are* looking for love, happiness, and fulfillment in all the wrong places. After teaching for fifteen years and interviewing thousands of people who appear to be living great lives, I can assure you this is true for almost everyone. Anyone with great success will more than likely tell you they needed more than their outside accomplishments in order to be happy, content, and fulfilled. Why? Because what our souls are hungry for is something we can't buy with accomplishment, money, or charm—something we can't even get from another human being. The truth is there is only one source of pure, unconditional, never-ending bliss, and that source resides inside of us. The only cost? Our devotion.

It may seem simplistic, but in this outer-driven world, it is easier to ignore the inner calling of your soul and buy into the extreme rationalizations of your human mind. Living a life of devotion to your highest self is a lifelong, daily pursuit. And it seems difficult only because you've been trained to look to the external world to get your needs met, to get the good feelings you're looking for. You think that if only you get the right body or the right relationship, if only you get that project finished or have all the love and money you want . . . you're sure there must be something in the external world that will finally deliver to you the satisfaction you crave deep within your soul.

Often, it takes a cracking open of your outer shell—some part of your life where you can't make sense of things, where you run into an obstacle you can't control or manipulate—to return you to the holy place within that can fuel and source a meaningful life. It is the events, circumstances, and experiences in the outer world that will ultimately expose the illusions that keep you stuck inside your human shell. You may have to lose your job or your money, experience the loss of a loved one or a betrayal, or become consumed by an out-of-control addiction to push past the closed doors of your ego's mind. I can assure you that all your challenges are there for one reason only: to turn you inward, and regardless of how you arrived here—through a desire to grow, a silent unhappiness, or a painful cracking open of the self—this cleanse bridges the gap between the internal and the external, so that you can return to your soul's deepest purpose by reconnecting to your divine essence.

When we are hungry for something to make us feel good about ourselves and we refuse to take care of our inner needs, we do stupid things. We get in repetitive patterns that we know will lead us nowhere. We succumb to our addictions, whether that means compulsively surfing the Internet and checking e-mail, shopping, viewing porn, eating, drinking, gambling, smoking, or spending. But most who suffer with deep feelings of emptiness know that there is nothing—and I mean nothing—that can fill that inner hole. Quick fixes and short-lived motivations just dig us deeper into the hole, leaving us more resigned in the present than we were in the past; hence the birth of the human chase.

Within you there is a hungry ghost that is always craving more, whether it's more love, money, respect, acknowledgment, or material possessions. No matter how much of these things you have, if you are emotionally deprived and spiritually impoverished, the hungry ghost takes over, and you find it impossible to feed its voracious appetite. This disowned part of yourself is never satisfied.

Ironically, though, when you allow yourself to connect to spirit, you want for very little because you're so rich and filled up inside. If all you ever prayed for, meditated on, and asked for was to open up to a deeper connection to this divine resource, everything that matches and vibrates on those higher levels of consciousness—including abundance, satisfaction, and a quiet mind—would come to you. But when you are disconnected from this source, *you hunger for anything that gives you the illusion that it will make you feel better.* The truth, though, is that there is only one solution to your inner hunger, only one way to satisfy the hungry ghost, and that is to fill it with love, with higher consciousness—to connect to all that you are and all that there is. When you are connected to your true essence, you feel blissfully content inside—one with your own soul and the spirit that sustains you. You're able to sail above the small, lonely feelings of your desperate heart that is searching for its divine counterpart. When you're connected to your soul's deeper purpose, you are able to bring to the world that which you long to give. When you're filled up inside by a power greater than yourself, you naturally feel love, compassion, and kindness for yourself and for others and are infused with the power and the confidence to be, do, and have that which best reflects and expresses your soul's highest potential.

When you are tapped in and connected from inside, you experience what the great twentieth-century novelist Franz

Kafka so gorgeously expressed when he wrote, "You don't even need to leave your room. Remain sitting at your table and listen. Don't even listen, simply wait. Don't even wait, just be still and solitary. The world will freely offer itself to you to be unmasked. It has no choice. It will roll in ecstasy at your feet." This is because when you have faith and trust in the divinity of every soul on this planet, you can see that God will answer the call of your individual soul—not in ego time but in divine time. And if you are quiet and centered enough to hear the voice of your own soul, you will be delivered a life beyond your wildest dreams.

Life truly is an amazing dance between the inner and the outer—a journey of your human needs and soul desires. You need the outer experience so that you will learn, grow, and evolve. But if you just go after the outer without tending to the inner, you end up empty and painfully disappointed. And if you just retreat to the inner world—unless you have chosen the life of a monk or happen to be a saint—you will likely experience isolation, loneliness, and lack. The powerful truth is that you are a child of the universe, a molecule of the divine spirit that orchestrates your greatest existence. And for you to truly experience a life of complete satisfaction, joy, and endless gratitude, you must accept that you are part of a much bigger game—a game in which if you win, I win. And if I win, you win. A game in which if I lose, you lose. And if you lose, I lose. A game in which the stakes are high and the winners are few, because you may be missing the basic rules of the game.

I am referring to life as a game not to trivialize it, but to bring you back to the realization that life was meant to be an adventure. When you approach the game of life from the perspective of the ego, you see it as a hard and arduous journey, and you end up feeling hurt, stuck, serious, and confused. When you look at life through the eyes of the soul, however, you see it as a playful dance, a school for your soul, something that is always changing and expanding. By following what I am calling "the rules of the game," you can take pleasure in all of life's expressions without getting stuck in any one experience. Following these rules is essential for getting the most value from the Consciousness Cleanse.

Preparing for
the Game

In order to play this divine game, you have to unhook tempo-
rarily from the outer world so you can tune in to the longing
of your soul. When you do, you can hear the whispers of
wisdom coming through the noisy, self-analyzing dialogue of
the mind. The powerful silence of an inner-directed life is
nourishment for your soul. By nature, your soul is soft, gentle,
loving, and kind. It is forgiving, peaceful, and humble. Confident and comforting in times of despair, your soul is strong,
focused, and determined in the mission called life.

Your soul neither brags nor boasts, because it is certain of its
power and grace. It never asks you to endure anything you
can't handle. It is made up of the sun and the rain, the wind and
the snow. It is attached to the leaves and the earth as well as

the moon and the stars. Although it has the quality of the "I," it gracefully dances with the "we," for it knows that all pairs of opposites are the same: heaven and hell, pain and pleasure, soft and hard, black and white, passive and aggressive, weak and strong, open and closed, stressed and relaxed, earthly and heavenly. It knows that you are either moving forward or going backward, strolling or running, accepting or rejecting, giving or receiving, organized or disheveled, controlling or surrendering, for you are a human being filled with both divine grace and human limitations. The game is this magical dance, a profound balance between the inner and the outer.

And it is your soul's journey to bring into balance all of what you are—the coexistence of opposites, the divine integration of the sum of all your parts. It is your soul's journey to enroll the ego in the quest for the ultimate victory—the evolution of your own individual consciousness. But the journey must begin by choosing between two forces: one has the power to lead you to new heights; the other can keep you pinned down to a past that is filled with limitation and dread. Don't be fooled. You're living either an ego-driven life or one that is soul-centered.

The soul discerns with a laserlike sharpness. The ego judges and rejects with disdain and aggressiveness. The soul takes responsibility. The ego blames and transfers responsibility. The soul moves through life with grace. The ego moves through life with recklessness, chaos, and drama. The soul feels good about who it is and what it wants and needs to sustain itself, to grow and evolve. The ego never has enough; it can never leave well enough alone or see beyond the current circumstances. It is entitled, confused, and feels stuck.

The ego tirelessly swims against the current, while the soul sits back and floats in the direction that life is moving in. You're either being guided by your soul or driven by your ego. At any time, you have access to either of these realities, and to all the experiences and emotions they bring with them.

You must understand that divine consciousness (your soul's journey) and human consciousness (your ego's path) coexist and are operating within you, all the time. Right now there is a full range of experience and emotion that is available to you. You can be burdened by fear, sadness, and suffering as you struggle against your perceived flaws, limitations, and outer obstacles. And the very next minute you can be filled with love, joy, and an exhilarating sense of freedom as you get hugged by your child, receive a bonus check from your employer, or are given a clean bill of health by your doctor. If you are not living in a way that supports your soul's highest expression, you'll inevitably fall prey to the devilish vibrations of your ego's lowest impulses.

The level of consciousness you choose to tune in to each moment of each day will determine the quality of your experience of the world. This is because everything in the universe is made up of energy, and this energy vibrates at different frequencies. Fear, resentment, and depression vibrate at a lower level and express your primal human tendencies, whereas love, joy, and appreciation are expressions of your higher self. When you are vibrating at a low level of consciousness, you can see only what isn't working; you focus on the negative—on your weaknesses, shortcomings, and unfulfilled desires. And when you're vibrating at a high level of consciousness, the world and everyone in it are as they should be. When residing in the higher realms of consciousness, you easily see possibilities and solutions—even if they look very different from what you would have expected. You are naturally in the flow, passionately determined to make the most of your life. You're at peace with who you are, even if there are changes to make and problems to solve.

When you're vibrating in harmony with your soul's highest emotions, you embark on an exhilarating ride to all that is good about life; when you give power to your ego's life-draining emotions, they take you on a depressing ride to the familiar territory of your problems, upsets, and dramas of the past. This is where you have a powerful choice to make. You can live in heaven, or you can suffer in hell. Heaven in this sense is a perfect state of divine consciousness. It's the experience of being completely present to all that is, all that you are, and all that you have to give. It is the experience of embracing and basking in the fullness of your divine nature; this is the soul's journey. And remember, you don't have to go very far to find heaven or hell. They're just one click away. People with hearts filled with love, peace, and compassion live in heaven. People who are consumed with fear, resentment, and guilt are experiencing a hell-like existence. Take a moment and remember a time when you've visited heaven

and now a time you were stuck in hell. Chances are you've encountered at least a few of life's greatest challenges. You can go
through those tough times kicking and screaming, whining and
complaining, or you can understand that you are experiencing
them for a very important reason—the evolution of your soul.

When you are present to this truth, you can choose the high
vibration of compassion during those moments when you're
overwhelmed by grief, loss, or fear. Compassion is one of the
highest states of consciousness that you can choose to assist
you in times of enormous pain. When you are riding with compassion, you will hear gentle, spirit-filled words that might say,
for example, "This, too, shall pass" or "God never gives you
more than you can handle." Compassion will whisper a greater
truth, like "No one deserves to be abused, but you will learn
from this and will be able to help other people when you're on
the other side of this challenge."

Maybe you will choose the vibration of faith, which offers
you the deep assurance that says, "You are never alone. I'm here
with you. God loves you. It's all going to be OK. You are over
the worst of it." When you choose a high vibration, you will be
wrapped in the arms of the Divine and resonate in the eternal
realms. But if you choose fear, martyrdom, anger, and hate, you
will more than likely live in a state of hell along with those
who have participated in your pain.

You can choose life-affirming behaviors that lift you up and
carry you to higher planes of consciousness, or you can give
up, be lazy, fall prey to the entitlement issues of your wounded

ego, and get swept into the darkness of your lowest impulses. When you choose to live in divine states of awareness, you will become privy to more and more levels of consciousness where guidance and information are infinite, where possibilities are endless, where support and safety are inexplicably present, where power and control cease to exist, and where love and surrender provide a magic-carpet ride to freedom.

RULE NO. 1:
UNHOOKING FROM THE OUTER WORLD

Throughout the years, I have witnessed thousands of people as they experience miraculous changes by unhooking (even for a little while) from their trancelike fixation on the external world and turning their attention inward, to a world without words, without limits, without wants and needs, a world without expectation and lack. I have experienced in myself, as well as in those I love and those I teach, the unprecedented leaps and successes that are birthed out of an inward-directed life.

I want you to imagine how this process of unhooking works. Every time you focus on an outer want or need, or on somebody else's business, it's like throwing a hook out and attaching yourself to the object of your attention. You can imagine these hooks as energetic bungee cords, transferring energy from your inner core to something outside of yourself. When you transfer your energy to something outside of your own inner world, you're literally giving away your peace, serenity, and power.

In order to attain the peace and tranquility of your highest self, you must take time to look and see what part of your life is controlling you, what part is taking you away from the tranquility of your inner sanctuary. If you're honest, you will see that on some days you have your attention on other people's dramas or maybe on an intense conversation you had with a co-worker days before. It could be that after splurging on your favorite meal, you obsess for hours, giving your power away to some food you ingested long ago. Or you obsess about money you lost in the stock market, a rude message left by your ex-husband or ex-wife, an opportunity you missed, an injustice you witnessed, or on some horrible experience that happened to you decades before. There are a million places where your energy might be right now, but only one place where you really need it, which is connected to the inner resource that has the power to guide you to love, success, and fulfillment. When you begin the process of unhooking, you can find literally hundreds of places where you have given your power away and drained your life force while guaranteeing the status quo.

How are you guaranteeing the status quo when you have hooks in the outer world? By directing far too much of the power and the energy that you need to re-create and reinvent your life toward all things outside of yourself. And to return to the place where you can hear the whispers of your soul's deepest desires and your highest truth, you need to be plugged in.

I can think of days, sometimes months, when I was obsessed with a thought or conversation about a situation in which I felt there was some abuse or injustice occurring. I've thrown hooks out because I wanted to be right or attain an ego-driven goal. And at the end of the day, I can see that I've given away thousands of hours of priceless energy. Anytime you give your power away to something outside yourself, you're actually disconnecting from your inner world, taking all that life-force energy and giving it away to the outer world—a world that is out of your control. This is the birth of powerlessness. Every time you throw hooks out, you're disconnecting from your power source. When you're disconnected, you lose your power, you lose your voice, you lose your ability to discern, and you trade off your precious inner resources for life-draining distractions and whims.

Now is the time to take back your energy, your power, and your peace. The cleanse will support you in tapping into your intuitive heart and opening up to new eyes, eyes that will guide you to everlasting love. It will assist you in becoming firmly rooted in greater realities. It's a process for learning how to access the divine presence and carry it with you wherever you go. It is the discovery of knowing you're never alone because you are one with a force of unlimited power and resources. And the great news is that you don't have to do anything "out there" to ensure this divine hook-up. But you do have to unhook from your daily to-do lists—not so that you will sink into a dark hole of inactivity and laziness, but so that you can reattach to what brings true meaning, happiness, and purpose to your life.

Unhooking guarantees you the ability to observe yourself and understand your life in ways that will leave you forever changed. It returns you to your roots, to your divine connection, so that you can see what stops you from being able to bask in, trust, know, and be surrounded by this infinite wisdom. Unhooking from the outer world supports you in seeing all the ways that you're controlled, manipulated, and used by your outer circumstances. It allows you to examine all that robs you of a soul-centered life.

Once you unhook from the outer world and bring that energy back into yourself, you discover unimaginable gifts: solutions to old problems, creative and visionary ideas, renewed energy, sparkling clarity, a sweeter connection to others, and exciting opportunities that you couldn't have seen coming. If you give yourself completely to this process for the next twenty-one days, new realities will open up for you. And I say this with utter certainty, because there are two amazing things about being human that I've come to understand over the many years that I've been writing, teaching, coaching, speaking around the world, and— maybe even more important—living a life filled with opportunities and challenges, good times and bad, limitations as well as limitless possibilities. This is what I know:

You are designed to reinvent and re-create yourself, over and over again. And, you are here—whether you want to acknowledge it or not; whether you even *know* it or not— for the evolution of your own soul.

And I imagine you can already feel that now, as you're reading these pages, because it is already happening—the turning inward, toward that awakened and vibrant level of consciousness that's available to you every moment of every day, *no matter what is going on out there.*

So, are you willing to unhook in order to reclaim your light? Are you ready to make your relationship with your most sacred self your number-one priority for the next twenty-one days? I can almost hear you saying, "Yes, I am ready. Yes, I am willing."

RULE NO. 2:
GIVING UP THE SELF YOU KNOW

Charles Dubois, the Belgian naturalist, said, "The important thing is this: to be able at any moment to sacrifice what we are for what we could become." So what does it take to let go of the self that you know? It takes tuning in to the calling of your deeper heart, the calling of your soul, and turning your life and will over to the care of the divine power within. It takes not knowing how and not being in control. The magic is found in understanding that coming to know God does not take place in your mind but rather in your heart. No matter what you may understand intellectually about God-consciousness, your mind can't take you there.

Your intellectual knowledge of God often prevents you from having the very real experience of God, because intellectual knowledge alone limits the possibility of something greater. When you allow your intellect to direct you rather than simply inform you, it limits what you can see, what you can do, what you can feel, and what you will experience. This is why contemplative practices are so important: they lift you out of your mind (funny—"out of your mind"). When you're out of your mind, you're free, you're peaceful, and you can see beyond your current reality. This is the life-changing shift: the ability to let go and open up to new realties over and over and over again and to break out of the illusion that what you see and what you know are right or real. To have this, you must be willing to be surprised.

Many of your long-held beliefs and much of your learned knowledge, while perhaps justified and reasonable, are limited. They may be perfectly correct in the confines of your emotional world or your intellectual understanding, but this is not what we are talking about here. In the realm of divine consciousness, most of what you consider to be facts about yourself are probably incorrect assumptions. What you know, and what you are certain about, are most likely the limiting beliefs that you adopted long ago, and they are what keep the door closed to your soul's highest wisdom. Each moment, you get to choose to look through the small, limited eyes of your human self or to be humble enough to take the quantum leap outside of what you may believe or know to be true. You must learn to trust that there is a future waiting that is beyond what you might be able to grasp at this moment.

The Grasper Effect

The promise of a larger life and a soul-inspired future is poignantly illustrated in *Grasper,* a beautiful children's story by Paul Owen Lewis.

Grasper, a sweet, young crab, lives near the rocks with many other fellow crabs. Together, they spend their days scavenging for bits of food and staying close to the place they think of as home. Then one day something peculiar happens to Grasper, as he begins to feel quite strange, as if he no longer fits inside his small body. Suddenly the world around him seems different. Trying to grasp what's happening, Grasper looks beside himself to see that his shell has split: now, instead of being on him, it is lying on the ground next to him. Grasper is shocked and scared to see a perfect silhouette of his crab body—arms, legs, eyes, and all—lying there beside him.

It isn't long before the other members of Grasper's tight-knit community of crabs have gathered in a circle around him. They explain to Grasper that his shell has just molted, and they caution him that weird things will begin to happen if he isn't careful. They tell Grasper that the period of time before his new shell hardens is very dangerous, and they warn him not to listen to the voices that will soon be filling his head. They tell him that he may want to explore places he's never seen before and may even be inclined to look beyond the rocks where they live. Grasper is perplexed.

Grasper hears what all the frightened crabs are telling him, and even though he wants desperately to fit in, belong, and please all his friends and family members, he is called by a higher voice and begins listening to and following his urge to explore the world outside of what he knows. Trusting his feelings, Grasper crawls out from behind the rocks where he has safely spent all of his life and ventures into new, unknown territory. All the while his friends are screaming, "Stop, Grasper! It's not safe out there!"

But when Grasper reaches the top of the rocks, he can't believe what he sees. Everything is colorful and bright. There are large, beautiful fish and lots of food to eat. It's a magical sight unlike any he has ever seen, and Grasper is filled with excitement. Then, coming out from behind a rock, Grasper comes face to face with a giant crab. It is the biggest crab Grasper has ever seen. When he asks the crab how he got so large, the crab explains to Grasper that the same thing will happen to him if he continues to grow and molt and allows himself to give up the life and the self that he knows. But Grasper can't believe this explanation because all the crabs he knows are as small as he is. The giant crab explains to Grasper that a crab grows only as large as the world he lives in, and as big as the heart inside him. He says, "You must have a big heart to live in a big world."

Grasper is mystified. He's been taught that to be safe in the world he must have a hard shell and a hard heart. But now he sees that if he wants to reach his full potential and grow into a giant crab, he will have to expand his horizons. Grasper will have to allow his heart to stay soft, for a hard heart can't grow.

Grasper is now faced with the biggest challenge of his life. His past is telling him that it would be safer to harden his heart and return to his familiar little home by the rocks. But the process of molting and softening has changed Grasper. He no longer wants just to survive. He longs to break free from the small world he has lived in and to swim out into the vast ocean to see who he will become.

This is the story of all of us. Like Grasper, when we are shedding an old identity, we naturally question who we *really* are, where we belong, and whether we'll still be lovable if we let go and allow the metamorphosis into a bigger, greater self to occur. We question whether we're going to be OK in the transition and are guaranteed a better life . . . for sure. Even if we can't bear living inside the small, uncomfortable confines of our outer shell, we have collected so much evidence that this is the safer choice, the smarter move to make. And yet the great paradox is that the profound process of letting go of the self we know is what gives us the strength to shake off the familiar shell of our past and place ourselves in the care of a power greater than ourselves. It is an act of faith, a commitment to our higher purpose, that gives us the confidence to leave the past behind and venture on to new territories.

The 21-Day Consciousness Cleanse supports you in a quickening of this process, helping you shed the layers of the past and open up to the grandeur of living in a larger world so that you can participate more consciously in the unfolding of your own divine story. It is the journey from your head to your heart; the journey from ego to soul, from thinking to feeling— the journey that addresses this fundamental truth: *your mind cannot and will not take you where your heart longs to go.*

So to win the game of your life, you must be willing to venture outside your mind—shed the skin of your past—and open up to the enormity of who you are. It is only when you accept your past that you can shed it and become open and malleable enough to make the journey out of the land that you've known, to return to your original sacred state of being. It is in this state of awareness that you can see the gift that you are and the blessings of your circumstances. Although this divine story unfolds uniquely for every one of us, I will assert that where your heart longs to go has everything to do with reconnecting with the inner resource that gives rise to the miracle you know as human life. But the caveat is that the real shift in consciousness, and the fulfillment of all that you desire, demands that you let go of the shore of the self you've known in order to embark on the hero's journey into the unknown. It requires you to choose daily to live a soul-centered, spirit-directed life—a life guided by a force greater than any self you know.

My Grasper Moment

It was my own cracking open that led me to search and explore beneath the surface of my own human shell. I was in my fourth drug-treatment center, and it was day ten of a twenty-eight-day program. By this time, I had suffered for over fifteen years with drug addiction and the underlying insecurities and self-loathing that birthed this painful pattern of behavior. I had been in and out of treatment centers before and could never seem to make it all the way through. It was always around the ten-day mark that I began to feel strong, willful, and convinced that I "had it." I don't know what I thought I had, but the ache that led me into the treatment center would fade away and be replaced by a desperate desire to get the hell out of there. But on this particular day, I was keenly aware of where my urge to escape would take me. It was no mystery, because it had happened so many times before. I would finagle my way out of the treatment-center door, claiming I was healed, had found enlightenment, and was now freed from my addiction. And then either hours, days, or weeks later I would be back in the same vicious cycle of filling my small body with drugs, chasing a feel-good moment, and then sinking back down into the depths of hell and hopelessness.

But on this particular morning I was finally able to see where the path of running away would lead me. And I knew without the shadow of a doubt that I couldn't do it one more time. I knew that if I ran away, I would either find myself back in the same place I was in or, worse, never make it back here alive. But even with this awareness, the urge to escape continued to well up inside of me, and the voices in my head became louder and louder: "Run, Debbie, run! Get out of here! You're not one of them. You don't need this. You don't need these people. You can do it alone! You're better than them." For hours I turned my attention to this inner voice and listened. I wanted to believe it. I wanted it to be the truth. But the harsh reality was that this voice had let me down so many times before. So maybe for the first time in my entire life, I decided to resist the urgings of this know-it-all voice and instead chose to explore the possibility that there was another way besides my way. I needed to explore this power that everyone kept talking about, this force that could give me some relief.

So I excused myself from the group-therapy session I was attending and proceeded down the dark, dingy corridor that led to the bathroom. I opened the door to the bathroom and was appalled by the smell of dried urine. The bathroom was a disgusting place. The stench was almost more than I could bear. The tiled floor and the grout that held the tiles together, which probably started out gray, were now black with mold. And even though I'm a bit of a clean freak, I forced myself into the room because at this point I was so filled with toxic emotions and so desperate for help that I decided to do the unthinkable: I got down on the floor on my hands and knees in a prayer position and began to pray. I asked God—or my higher power, as they called it—to come to me, to help me, to rescue me from my pain and my own self-destruction. My body was trembling, and tears were rolling down my cheeks. I was desperate for help, for understanding, and for salvation. And although I had attended synagogue all my life, attended many 12-Step meetings, and heard all types of people talk about God, for me God was nothing more than a man in the sky, a concept in my mind that brought me neither comfort, peace of mind, nor faith. The actual experience of God, spirit, or divine consciousness did not exist for me.

So for a few minutes, I listened to the ranting in my head about how stupid this was, how disgusted I was to be here, and how embarrassed I felt begging some power I didn't even believe in to help me. I felt angry at God, at my parents, and at all those who had hurt me, believing that if it weren't for all of them I wouldn't be here, literally experiencing an all-time low. I tried to convince myself that I could get up and leave, but my fear that I would die if I ran away had led me here, and now it urged me to stay.

I thought back to the day before I entered this treatment center. I was living in an apartment in North Miami Beach, Florida. I owned a thriving clothing store in a prestigious mall and had a powerful business partner who had given me the opportunity of a lifetime. From the outside, it looked like I had it all as I drove around in my white Porsche convertible, wore the hippest clothes, hung out with the coolest people, and partied in the Miami nightlife until the wee hours. Certainly I had gotten the mask of my outer shell to look just right. I was the girl who had it all: money, success, opportunities, friendships, and the world at my fingertips. But what most people who knew me didn't know was that in the quietness of my own inner world, I hated myself. I hated my superficial life. I hated my insecurities and my fear. I hated the emptiness that taunted me day in and day out. I was angry, judgmental, confused, and out of control. I was tired, desperate, and lonely, and the only thing that ever took away or at least quieted that noisy little voice of my pain was the carefully selected mixture of drugs that I would faithfully consume each day.

The truth was that the drugs had stopped working long ago. And although I could barely endure the thought of having to live without them, I knew I wouldn't live much longer with them. Just two weeks earlier I had scored a bottle of a thousand Percodans from a girl I had befriended who worked in a pharmacy. When I met her, I thought I had struck gold. She was going to be the answer to my dreams and the solution to the countless hours I spent trying to round up enough drugs to get me through each week. But here on this dark day, this day of reckoning, even that bottle was empty. It startled me. It wasn't that I had never experienced an empty bottle before, but there had been a thousand pills in this big, brown glass pharmaceutical bottle, and less than fourteen days later they were gone. I now needed to take at least ten Percodans at a time to catch a feel-good moment, when just a few years earlier I had needed only one. The bag of cocaine that I dipped the ends of my cigarettes in to accompany my Percodan high was empty as well.

Here I was face-to-face with an out-of-control, all-consuming drug addiction, surrounded by ashtrays, empty cartons of Salems, and my bottle of ten-milligram Valium that I used to begin each day. I was obsessed with trying to figure out how my life had come to this. I seemed to be a genius at rationalizing, denying, lying, and making up excuses for my bad behavior, but on this day, with the empty bottle in hand, I knew in the depth of my soul that I just couldn't go on living like this. I couldn't pretend that I was OK for one more day. The scene was still vivid in my mind. All my clothes were thrown all over my room as I ransacked every drawer looking for pills that I might have hidden and dollar bills that might still contain some residue of cocaine. My purses were scattered across my closet floor as I searched tirelessly, knowing there must be something, some residue, somewhere. All the plastic bottles in my bathroom that had held my pills were now uncapped and lying on the marble countertop.

As I continued frantically searching, I felt the desperation, the fear, the powerlessness of needing a fix and being unable to find one. I could have picked up the phone, but I was too ashamed and humiliated to call even my drug dealers. No one could consume this amount of drugs in such a short time. I was mortified and filled with shame when I knew that no cute leather dress or outrageous dangling earrings could hide the pathetic nature of this scene. Even my drug dealers would know what a real loser I was. And the moment I realized that I was embarrassed of myself in the face of people whom I considered to be the scum of the earth, I knew there were no other options. I had to reach out once again and get some help. The very fact that I thought I was going to die was probably second to the sickening feeling of being a blown-out drug addict—the poor little rich girl. Here I was with everything, and yet I had nothing, because I had lost the only things that mattered: the connection to myself, and the divine resource I now call God.

After recalling this desperate and painful scene, my mind snapped back into the present moment, and I once again became aware of the cold tiles underneath me. There, on my hands and knees, not knowing what else to do, I began reciting the Serenity Prayer, which I had recently learned:

> God, grant me the serenity
> To accept the things I cannot change;
> Courage to change the things I can;
> And wisdom to know the difference.

I focused on each phrase, because I was desperate for a moment of inner peace. More than anything in the world, I just wanted a few minutes of quiet inside my noisy mind. I whispered the words just loud enough so I could hear them over and over and over again: "God, grant me courage to change." I wanted to change; I needed to change, or I was going to kill myself. I was begging and crying hysterically. With my head in my hands, I sobbed uncontrollably, rocking my body from side to side, trying to soothe my broken heart, until suddenly I realized that something inside of me had shifted: a calm had come over me, a silence that was palpable. In asking God, this higher power, to enter my awareness, something inside of me had opened up and relaxed. Slowly, the stress in my body and the screaming voice in my mind subsided, and peace enveloped my entire being. Even the filthy, disgusting bathroom floor didn't look so bad. There was a release, a letting go, a clarity, an expansiveness, but most important, there was some hope. My God, I had hope. Just what my soul needed most.

That morning I knew I had experienced something very important, significant . . . life-changing. Even though I didn't know what it was exactly, I did know that I was lifted out of the pain of my emotional body, at least for the time being, and brought into the precious present. I knew then that I could at least make it through another day. And at that point, one more day was all I really needed. I was spontaneously filled with a deep inner knowing that not only could I survive, but I would get through this dark night of the soul and be able to thrive when I was released from this perceived hellhole. And all I wanted to do was run back into my group session and shout out to my fellow addicts, "I can do it! We can do it! And guess what, there really is a power greater than ourselves that can help."

I share this experience on the bathroom floor of the West Palm Beach Institute because it was the defining moment when I discovered that a power greater than the self that I knew existed. It was in this moment that I began to heal and transform my inner world and form a deep, loving relationship with the power that I now know as God. It was my day, my miracle, my choice point. And every day for the next eighteen days, I made the choice to find my way back into that bathroom, which had become my holy sanctuary—a place where I could reconnect with the all-loving presence that had delivered me access to the higher aspect of myself and this inner resource that could shift a moment of pain to a moment of awakening. Through this daily ritual of prayer, I found the strength to finally make it through all twenty-eight days of treatment. On one warm Florida day nearly twenty-six years ago, I walked out of my last treatment center, knowing that I had tapped into a power and a resource that could remove obstacles, change people's perceptions of the world and their lives, and lead me to a future I couldn't even fathom. That day, I knew with every fiber of my being that I needed to further explore, understand, and, more important, devote my life to finding and knowing God.

As I continued my healing process and resumed my life, I was consumed by the need to understand how this shift had occurred. Why this time did I find the strength I had failed to find so many times before? How did I go from feeling deep pain, agony, and despair to experiencing peace, joy, and contentment? How could I feel so alone and separate one moment, and a moment later feel completely connected, one with all that is, seen and unseen? How did I go from seeing the world through the self-centered eyes of my wounded ego to glimpsing the unbelievable intricacies and possibilities of my inner life?

To this day, I remain awed and fascinated by what's available to every one of us when we reconnect to our soul's deepest desires. The quest to understand this powerful source has led me on a long, unbelievable journey, from the depths of darkness and despair to unimaginable moments of light, love, creativity, and joy. And the unquenchable desire of my soul to have all of my questions answered and the mystery of unseen powers revealed is ultimately what has led me to the 21-Day Consciousness Cleanse . . . and the return to light that it promises.

Leaving my shell behind—which included many friends, behaviors, and habits; a plethora of negative beliefs and false assumptions; and an army of grudges and resentments—has allowed me to hear and follow the longing of my soul's deepest purpose. My soul knew I would be a teacher, writer, and friend to many. My soul knew I had all the ingredients to express my God-given wisdom to others and to develop myself into a woman who now considers herself an order-taker. *Who is my master?* you might ask. My master is a power I've never seen but that I've experienced, a power that is here to give and not to get, to offer rather than push; a power that seeks goodness but doesn't judge darkness. My master is a loving presence that guides me to continually take risks, to share my deepest pain as well as my greatest joy; a master who is always guiding me toward the light of my precious soul even when I can't understand where we are going, a master who urges me to make better choices even when my human needs are calling me to an earthly desire.

RULE NO. 3:
THE WILLINGNESS TO SHIFT

What happened on the bathroom floor that day, I now know, is what's called a *shift in consciousness*. And it took a cracking open of the self I knew to facilitate this shift. For a few moments, I was lifted out of the pain of my emotional body and the insanity of my tumultuous mind and transported into a place that is all loving, all knowing, quiet, secure, and relaxed. I had entered the "holy land" where God-consciousness resides. In just a few moments—that's all it took—I was able to open to a place inside myself that literally had the power to shift and redirect my entire life.

This shift, available to any of us at any time, requires nothing more than for us to slip out of our own separate human drama and reconnect with the divine resource that resides within. We've all heard the phrase "Ask and you shall receive." Well, it's true, because our willingness to ask is what opens the door for us to receive the love and guidance of our higher self. Our willingness to resign as general manager of the universe and admit that we do not know everything unhooks us from the stagnant trance of our own individual, separate realities. And once we are able to own up to this truth and concede that we can't do this on our own, the lower aspects of ourselves settle down and the door to the higher realms opens. This is what allows for the shift to occur.

You can choose to take the difficult road of doing it your way—all alone, as director and solitary leader—or surrender to a higher will and live in partnership with the greater whole. If you choose the latter, you must be willing for your heart to remain open as you extend the invitation to which God will gracefully respond. When divine consciousness enters, the shift occurs and you will be engulfed by what will feel like the greatest love imaginable—a love in which your soul realigns with your spirit and they meet together as one.

As you make the internal space for God to enter, you open up to a larger, more soul-filled reality than the one you are currently living in. The God that I speak of is not an all-powerful presence that lives outside of you, but rather a universal force that resonates in the core of your being, connecting you to all that is and all that will be. It's an all-encompassing energy that is creative, powerful, and wise—a force that is sometimes referred to as spirit, love, the divine universal consciousness, or our golden essence. It is known by many names, and there are countless paths that can lead you to reconnect with the powerful presence that resides within you. This force has the power to light you up from the inside, but to reconnect with it, you need the humility to step outside of the grandiosity of your limited, separate self and express an honest and humble desire to know this spiritual power.

To know your golden essence is to chip away at your external self and be willing to rediscover yourself in the highest and purest form. It is to glimpse the part of you that exists beyond your limitations, beyond your stories, beyond your doubts, fears, and insecurities, and beyond your critical mind. Even though this force is unseen, when you join together with it, when your thoughts, beliefs, and feelings are aligned with it, you can feel it. It's palpable. God is a very real vibration that exists. You can feel it pulsating through your body. You can feel it through the love in your heart and the satisfaction of your soul. When you are fully immersed in this divine presence, you want for nothing, because you have everything. By cleansing your consciousness of the debris of the past, you open yourself more and more to the high vibration of infinite wisdom and divine oneness. It is in this state that you return to wholeness, which is exactly what you are at the deepest level.

Emmet Fox, the divinely inspired twentieth-century minister, writer, and mystic, tells us, "This state of mind is really the one thing that is worth possessing, for having that, one has it all; and lacking that, he has nothing." To reach this state is the real objective of the Consciousness Cleanse. In this higher state of being, you know you are protected, guided, and deeply loved. When the divine is present, you have faith in your innate ability to heal trauma, heartache, and dis-ease. You have faith in your power to make negative emotions and the other day-to-day problems of life disappear, evaporate, as a higher knowing emerges. Anywhere there is unwanted dis-ease, whether it is dis-ease in your body or in your mind, you will discover that spirit is missing from these areas of your life. However, when you are one with the creative force of the universe, aligned with your golden essence and your soul's higher purpose, you are gifted with the willingness to step further into the unknown and trust that you are part of a grander play. When you are willing to *not* know, to not understand, to not have it all figured out, to not be in charge, to not have life go the way you think it should go—to not be playwright, director, actor, and stagehand—then miracles can happen. Life can surprise you only when you are willing to be surprised, when you are willing to open your eyes in the morning and have a brand-new day emerge. Not a day like yesterday. Not a day that you expect. Not a day when you systematically behave in the same old ways, think the same repetitive thoughts, and create the same expected outcomes. A day when you are surprised by the magic of your consciousness, by your deeper desire to give and love; surprised by your desire to take responsibility for your past and your future; surprised by your deeper desire to live for today rather than dwell in the fantasy of a future that is not here yet. When you are completely surprised by what you are willing to give up and what you crave to take on, you will experience the miracle of miracles: a soul reborn. This doesn't have to happen just once. It can happen each day as you escape the suffocation of your soul's dreams and transcend the malignancy of middle age.

When you embrace the dream your soul holds for you, and when you allow your divine heart to be your director and guide, you will be able to receive the many gifts that are waiting for you to open and enjoy—extraordinary realities that might now seem unattainable. For most, these gifts do indeed show up like miracles. But let me remind you that your ego probably doesn't like miracles, because miracles are an expression of a greater reality, a reality beyond your limitations. Miracles are truly nothing more than occurrences that are outside the realm of what you once believed to be possible. So for a miracle to happen (which inside your ego structure can happen only if you are willing to be wrong about what you know, which pisses the ego off more than anything), you must give up your righteous positions and limiting beliefs and challenge what you believe to be the truth of your life. The Consciousness Cleanse will help you do this. By enrolling your ego in this mission and engaging with it in fresh, new ways over these twenty-one days, it just might surrender control so that these surprising and beautiful new realities can emerge. In this way, the Consciousness Cleanse is a holy invitation to forces seen and unseen to guide and support you, and to orchestrate miracles on your behalf.

RULE NO. 4:
GOD FIRST

I'm often asked why it's so difficult to maintain a high level of peace, serenity, and gratitude: "Why can't this whole process of being happy and living in a state of unlimited possibility be easier?" There are many answers to this poignant question. But this is what you need to remember: Your ego's job is to create an outer shell so that you can know yourself as a unique, individual expression. Your ego is your unique human expression.

But if you are not aware of the workings of the ego, it will take over your entire consciousness like a cancerous tumor. When you remain blindly rooted inside your ego structure, your connection to your higher power is clouded over. It still exists, but the channel through which you can experience it becomes blocked by the confines of your ego's wall, the constrictions of your ego's grasp.

In other words, it is the outer persona, the shell of your human ego, that blinds you from seeing this very resource hidden within.

I love the acronym for ego: "Easing God Out." When you are completely identified with the shell of your individual self, your ego, you are blind to this divine state of consciousness, this light that is sometimes called God. This is one of life's great paradoxes, because to be a human being is to have an outer shell, an ego presence. You need your ego's persona in order to distinguish yourself from others. It's only when you fail to recognize that your outer shell is just one aspect of who you are that you shut the door on God's light. You ease God out. Then the channel through which you experience God's love becomes closed and you're trapped inside your ego's shell, which offers only a limited perspective. When you're inside your ego, you can think about God and talk about God, but you can't feel or experience God's presence. And it's not until you can acknowledge this divine resource that you will truly know and see yourself as the gods and goddesses that you are. When you're aware of the gold within, you're connected to this force of light. Then you can bring conscious awareness, love, and compassion to your ego's insatiable needs. This is what allows you to open up, to chip away at your outer shell. The more divine light and love you let in, the more deeply you will feel your connection with the divine force. It is easy to make the ego wrong and label it the "black sheep" of the family. But it's not. Your outer shell plays a vital role in the expression of your individual gifts. So for you to truly live in this world—not as a secluded monk but as a high-functioning human being—your ego just needs a gentle (or not so gentle) reminder that its function is to go out and gather the experience and wisdom it needs to fulfill your soul's calling. Part of the experience is for you to muster up the courage and strength to go beyond your families' and ancestors' limitations and hear the voice of your soul even if your ego begs you to accept mediocrity over excellence. Even though your ego may not remember its divine function, its deepest desire is to be one, reunited with the power and force that is greater than itself.

So how can we ensure this oneness? We move our soul's evolution to the forefront and make it the goal of the game. We remind ourselves that the big win is not *he who dies with the most toys* but rather *he who has delivered his soul's greatest purpose to the world*. The only way to ensure victory over our human operating system is to put our soul's purpose first. To do this we must presence God first in the morning, before we get out of bed, before we eat a meal or drink a glass of water; God before we work, before we make a phone call, before we communicate with a co-worker or our children, before we go to bed at night, before we create something, and before we ask for anything.

If we don't put God first, we will be run over by the demands of our outdated persona, which wants to fill the eternal hole with material things and other people's love and approval. We must be humble enough to remember that this is the poorest substitute in the world for real, unimaginable love. If we are always trying to mix saccharin or some other human-made chemical with our pure, essential self, thinking that it will satisfy our taste for divine sweetness, we will never know divine love. Substitutions will never suffice. The hole inside is looking to be filled. It is the hole of a lost soul aimlessly trying to be seen and heard, an innocent child helplessly watching the next human car wreck. But it is only with the purest of hearts—and the holiness of this untapped divine resource—that the soul can heal and the human heart can sing with joy as it experiences the fullness and satisfaction of a fully expressed life.

Reclaiming your light and returning to your holy essence is a process of giving up who you are, what you believe, and what you expect so that you can discover the spirit in you that is indefinable, unlimited, and spectacular. And when you are in the presence of this spirit, you will no longer have to try to be someone you're not. You won't have to try to be good enough, smart enough, thin enough, rich enough, funny enough, special enough, interesting enough, caring enough, important enough, or selfless enough. You just get to be whoever you authentically are in that moment. You won't want the light; you'll

be the light. You will no longer seek the beloved; you will
know that you are the beloved.

RULE NO. 5:
EXPANDING YOUR CONTAINER

We are here to open ourselves up to greater dimensions of reality so that we may make peace with God, self, and others.
There is no better way than God's way. We can try and do and
take and challenge, but we will never know pure unadulterated
love until we look and feel through the eyes and heart of our
eternal essence and access our soul's inner voice. No one and
nothing can propel us to the heights we yearn to attain except
this divine power. No one thing (sex, drugs, shopping, achieve-
ment, or food) can fill the hole in our soul—because the hole is
so huge. No man, woman, or thing (success, money, or accomplishments) is big enough to fill this measureless space. That is
why so many try and fail: they are trying to fill a hole as big as
the Atlantic Ocean. And even a billion dollars dropped into a
body of water that large would disappear in seconds. So try as
we might, we will ultimately fail, because no outer thing—and
I mean *nothing*—can fill this bottomless hole.

We may ask ourselves, *If there is an infinite source of love, wisdom,*
and guidance to tap into at every moment of our lives, why don't we dip in
and take our share? It's as if we have forgotten how or forgotten
that this is our birthright. And even when the yearning for our
divine connection is very great, it's clear that we can draw forth

from this limitless source only as much as we can contain—or are willing to hold—in our own individual consciousness. In this case, it is because God won't give us more than we can handle. In essence, we can't tap into the power that has the ability to get us through the most difficult times and clear away the most daunting obstacles to our true fulfillment and ongoing success unless we make room for it—and we are the only ones who can do this. It is our responsibility to become a clear, vast container into which this divine infinite source can flow through us.

In Emmet Fox's book *Power Through Constructive Thinking* (which I've carried around with me for the last twenty years), the author proclaims:

> As far as God is concerned, our supply of Divine Energy is, of course, absolutely unlimited; there is no check of any kind upon the amount of it that we can appropriate, or, therefore, upon the things that we can do or be with it. Yet, for practical purposes, it remains that any given time you can draw from the inexhaustible Source only in accordance with the measure of your understanding.

Fox goes on to give us the following amazing image. Imagine going to the shore of the ocean with a small pitcher in your hand and leaning down and filling it up. Notice that you can hold only the amount of water that is in direct correlation to the size of the container you're using. If you've brought only a pint jar, you're not going to get a gallon. The point Fox is making is this: most of us are going to the shore of this inexhaustible resource with a small pitcher in our hands when what we need to live our highest potential is to have access to the whole body of water . . . this wealth of infinite wisdom and divine power. Just as the deep blue ocean is boundless and immeasurable, so is our divine resource. And when it comes to dipping into this infinite reservoir, we can use a container the size of a pint, a quart, a gallon, or even a water tank if we're willing. But what is certain is that we can take in only the amount of water that's in accordance with the size of the container. The Consciousness Cleanse is a holy process for you to use to expand your container.

Settling for less is too often what we do in our relationship to spiritual power. The reason we don't have access to all of it is simply that we've made no room for it within ourselves. We fill the sacred vessel of our consciousness with so many distractions and so much noise that we can't even hear the whispers of our intuitive heart or see the signs and signals that are meant to guide us, protect us, and ensure that we are thriving. We don't have the wherewithal or the will to truly embrace the present, because we haven't fully digested the past. We're maxed out. We're so busy, we can't even hear ourselves think, let alone hear the voice of our own soul. Even when we're warned by a gut reaction to make a different choice or take a different path, most of us will choose to ignore the voice of our higher guidance and do what seems easiest at the moment.

If we are not committed to growing, evolving, and living our best life, we will inevitably search for and find outer fixes—some form of instant gratification to numb our pain and keep us in a state of denial so that we can forget about our unfulfilled dreams. We all have the right to stay comfortably numb, with our soul's gifts hidden from ourselves and the world. Instant gratification is always an option if we aren't ready to listen to the voice of our souls or do the work necessary to clear away the toxic residue of our past and return to our highest mission. Most of us have found ourselves off our path more than once, being driven to make impulsive decisions that have led us away from our dreams and down a long, dark road to nowhere. If we refuse to take time to care for our interior world, to nourish and honor our holiest selves, we will be thwarted in our best intentions and hijacked by our automatic programming, which, by the way, is almost always influenced by the dark moments of our past and is in opposition to reaching our highest expression.

If you don't periodically detoxify your mind through a Consciousness Cleanse, you can think affirming thoughts and read uplifting books all day long, but these new thoughts can't actually penetrate into your awareness because it is already filled to the brim. There is no more room, so your mind rejects the new thoughts and cancels them out because there are other beliefs that are in opposition to what you're trying to put in. For example, imagine that you've made a vision map for the future you want to create, and it is loaded with images and words that all say, "I am successful." Your vision map depicts a life in which you have a lot money in the bank and a great job, you're well-respected, and you're thoroughly enjoying the fruits of your labor. With a candle lit next to your new vision map, you meditate on it, pray about it, and dwell in it. But in a short time you begin to get frustrated and impatient, wondering why your success isn't immediately forthcoming. What you can't see is that "I am successful" can't take root when what is already taking up space in your consciousness is an old belief that you've been holding for the past twenty-five years: "I'm a failure." You first have to evict "I'm a failure" in order to make room for "I'm a success." Then your success can move in and you will begin to flourish.

Another example of an opposing belief is one that many people can relate to. Let's say that you dream of having a life-long intimate relationship with a wonderful man but your father left you when you were three years old. At that tender age, you subconsciously decided you were unlovable or that love is painful. Your unformed psyche scrambled to make sense of why daddy would leave, and you came to the painful conclusion that you were to blame. And so for the past thirty-five years, "unlovable" has taken up all the room and is squatting in every square foot of your consciousness. This is why so many people are frustrated and resigned after years of doing affirmations to no avail. Your ultimate goal must be to evict all squatters and for this, you must accept that the past is the past so that you can cleanse your consciousness.

Once your mind is still and quiet, once it is relieved of the turbulence of all your toxic thoughts, you open up the space, the pure fertile ground, to encode your consciousness with new ways of being, new thoughts and beliefs, and thrilling futures. In the same way that cleansing your physical body of accumulated impurities allows you to better absorb nutrients from the food you eat, cleansing your consciousness of your past experiences and outdated thoughts—as well as of your paralyzing feelings of grief, regret, and anger—allows you to tap into a well of life-affirming thoughts, ideas, and emotional states.

The Promise

You are about to embark on a twenty-one-day journey of detoxification and spiritual renewal that promises to radically and permanently alter both the quality and the direction of your life. The Consciousness Cleanse is a deep soul cleansing that will support you in clearing out everything that stands in opposition to your true magnificence and the unlimited expression of your highest self. It is designed to deliver incredible, measurable, and tangible results that will alter the way you see yourself, others, and the world. It is designed to help you release the old and make room for the new. As each day builds upon the next, you will gain a palpable experience of deep peace—a profound knowing, pulsating in every cell of your being, that you are worthy of finding and living your soul's deepest passion. You will discover how you can love yourself even when things aren't turning out your way; how you can love yourself even when you've made poor choices or when you failed to create the boundaries needed to protect yourself. You'll discover how you can be kind to yourself even when you're fat and broke. (Yes, you can.) You'll discover how you can love yourself even when your husband or wife has left you and your kids aren't speaking to you. You'll learn how to be compassionate to yourself when you feel flawed or defeated and when you feel like you've missed your calling. You'll discover how you can love yourself even when you're scared to death. In the process of the cleanse, you will learn to love all of yourself, knowing that there is no other love that is more important.

So even though you were born into unique circumstances within a particular family, with a particular set of strengths and challenges, blessings, shortcomings, and opportunities, it is your holy work, your job, to deeply love, honor, and respect the precious self that you are, the soul that only you hold. There is nothing else for you to do but to truly love and nourish the emotionally and spiritually starved parts of you that are crying out for your attention. This is the antidote, the answer, and the solution out of which all divine realizations are born.

The Consciousness Cleanse presents you with a priceless opportunity to release anything other than the frequency of love, compassion, kindness, tenderness, and possibility. With ease and effortlessness, you will withdraw your attention from the outer world and open up to the higher realms that are available within. In twenty-one days' time, you will see the radiance of your spirit restored as you bask in the excitement of a life yet to be lived.

The Process

In the weeks to come, you will have the extraordinary opportunity to purify the soil of your consciousness. As a gardener must till the soil of his garden before it can nourish and sustain new life, the Consciousness Cleanse will give you the opportunity to clear out the overgrown weeds of your past—the negative thinking, turbulent emotions, false assumptions, outdated beliefs, unresolved incidents, and limiting thought forms—that have taken root inside your mind. In the first seven days you will expose the beliefs and assumptions that have disconnected you from your holiest self and diluted the potency and effectiveness of your soul's highest expression. As you clear away the roots of your past, you will find yourself more deeply rooted in the present moment, where all of your power lies. As you unhook, release, and detoxify, you will be liberated from confusion, fear, guilt, and self-doubt. Cleansing the past will open up new realms of awareness, provide a window into your soul's passion, and usher you into the experience of emotional freedom and spiritual liberation.

Because the Consciousness Cleanse is intended to create radical breakthroughs, it begins powerfully. In the first seven days, you'll be asked to go straight for the life-changing release of everything that has depleted your vitality and held you back. Until you release these old emotions—your hardened grief, bitter resentments, deadening regrets, and seriously out-dated beliefs—you can't allow all of the power, wisdom, and light of your higher self. When tapped, this healing resource is yours for the taking and costs nothing to access. You need only clear a space and extend an invitation, and it will come flood-ing in. As you release the toxic buildup from your past, you naturally and effortlessly make room for this power to source you, to guide you, and to fuel you with the passion to live a life you love.

This powerful resource can be accessed only in the present moment. It isn't anything that lives out there in the future; it is available right now as you open yourself up to this moment in time. So during the next seven days of the cleanse, standing in the present, you'll take an honest look at where—and who— you are today. You'll observe everything you're doing and notice what is and what is *not* working. You will come to under-stand that the present moment is *the* pivotal point of power . . . the only place where you have a 360-degree relationship with your life. It's where you get to choose, moment by moment, how to relate to your past and your future. Standing firmly inside the present moment, you get to decide how much divine power you will claim as your own and how you will treat and respond to the calling of your soul.

The last phase of the cleanse will bring you some of the most exhilarating insights of your life. In this holy phase, you will have the opportunity to look into the future and see who you want to be from this day forward. How are you meant to manifest the glory of God? What internal and external structures does your soul need to ensure that you will actualize the potential that is yours to express? What daily rituals, prayers, practices, and behaviors will deliver you each day into the arms of the greatest power in the universe?

This twenty-one-day journey will bring a depth of exploration that may surprise you. You will no doubt encounter the Hungry Ghost that has kept you addicted to all manner of false comforts; you'll confront your faithlessness in the areas where you're failing; and you'll cultivate an astonishing and respectful relationship with your ego. You will loosen and finally assimilate the undigested, toxic thoughts and emotions that have built up over time, allowing you to finally let go of the past and align yourself with the divine force that will give you the ride of your life. As you plant the seeds of your soul's desires, you will encode your consciousness with purpose, meaning, and passion and evoke a spiritual resonance of love, peace, kindness, and tenderness. These high states of being will profoundly affect how you treat yourself, others, and the world.

As you navigate through the three phases of the cleanse, know that you will be bathed in a daily spiritual practice of meditation, contemplation, prayer, journaling, and other practices of self-discovery to help you venture beyond your mind, turn inward, and attune your awareness to the heart of God. In this state of deep stillness and intimate communion, you will rise above the mundane, transcend your moods, release your fears and anxieties, and reconnect with your highest self. You will rid yourself of self-doubt and self-condemnation, cleanse your subconscious mind, and make room in your heart for peace, health, and an abundance of happy times.

As you listen more deeply to the voice of your soul's unique desires, you will develop and strengthen your innate capacity to elevate yourself, at any moment, from the gravitational pull of stressful situations—whether it's a hurtful exchange with a loved one, a difficult circumstance at work, or a horrible act of violence that takes place in the world. You'll access the inner resource that connects you with your inner wisdom, enabling you to navigate your way out of the darkness of your own negative feelings and into the light of your higher self. As you ask the universe to be your partner and guide on the path to wholeness, you will find that this loving force is more than willing to take you by the hand and be your trusted companion. This awareness will leave you optimistic—even ecstatic— about what lies ahead.

As the field of your consciousness becomes translucent and pure, it will once again sustain healthy thoughts, loving feelings, brilliant ideas, and unlimited possibilities. By cultivating the fertile terrain of your own inner world, you enter the promised land of milk and honey, where the nourishment of mother's milk and the sweetness of appreciation are abundantly available. Here, the experience of love, contentment, and compassion can blossom. Your inner world—once overgrown and encumbered with painful regrets, judgments, and self-criticism—is now transformed into a place of pristine tranquility that perfectly reflects the mind of God.

The Preparation

To get everything out of the Consciousness Cleanse that you desire, preparation is crucial. After almost two decades of leading transformational workshops and training programs, I'm clear that the right preparation is imperative and will determine the results that you achieve. The care you bring to the setup of the cleanse will support the entire process and dictate either the ease of the process or the struggle that you may experience along the way. By making preparations that are tailored to your unique needs, you can dramatically increase the effectiveness of the cleanse.

The first step in preparing for your Consciousness Cleanse is to declare this as a holy time for yourself, a time for reflection and refueling, a time to cleanse the field of your inner world so it is capable of sustaining and nourishing your deepest and most heartfelt desires. Like a three-week exotic meditation retreat, this is an opportunity to unravel and unhook from the outer world and to return to the sanctuary that exists within. To do this, you must commit to becoming the keeper of your own inner flame.

Within you there exists an internal flame that is the keeper of your vitality and the guardian of your life force. The ancient Vedic text known as the Rig Veda describes this as the fire in the belly, an internal flame that has the power to digest what is no longer needed and to ward off pathogens, whether in the mind, the body, or the spirit. This internal flame guards and protects your essence as it illumines the path back to your highest self.

Every choice you make either adds to this force, making it stronger, igniting and feeding your flame, or diminishes the force, dampening your internal flame and reducing both your essence and your vitality. When your internal flame burns brightly, you are aligned with your soul's highest purpose and you feel strong, powerful, and confident. You have the strength and courage to ask—clearly and truthfully—for what you need, and you have the humility to listen to the wisdom that arises from within. A healthy, strong flame fills your mind with the inspiration to conceive big dreams and energizes your body with the stamina to pursue them. When you pay attention to your internal fire, providing it with the love, care, and compassion it craves, you will see with clarity and act with courage and focus. A strong flame propels you into the sanctuary of higher states of consciousness, where self-love and emotional freedom reside.

But if you deprive your flame of the food it hungers for, you easily fall prey to fear, worry, and self-doubt. When your flame is low, you are vulnerable to repeating behaviors from your past and perpetuating beliefs that imprison you behind walls of limitation. When your flame has been ignored, you hunger for things outside yourself to make you feel better. You seek nourishment from external achievements rather than from the inner source that gives you life. Skepticism and cynicism are the signs of a weak flame as you give credence to that which isn't working rather than celebrate what is.

A flame that is well nourished and thriving holds all the power of a sea of angels, lifting you above the seductive temptations of the past and securing you in the wisdom and guidance of your divine source. But, like any fire, your internal flame must be looked after and protected. To keep it burning brightly, you must honor and care for it, listen to it, tend to it, and nourish it. You are the keeper of your soul, and it is your job to do whatever is necessary to protect your flame from weakening. Without this level of attention and awareness, you will more than likely continue to repeat the patterns of the past, recycle the same life-draining thoughts and behaviors, and ultimately accumulate more toxicity in your mind.

To clear your consciousness so that the light of a new day can arise, you must become keenly present to the condition of your internal world and the strength of the fire within your soul. For the next twenty-one days, you will give your unwavering attention to different facets of your inner flame to see what is needed to build it into a roaring fire—to stoke the embers that are longing to burn brightly and to clear away anything that threatens its extinction. During the first seven days of the cleanse, as you're focused on making peace with the past, you'll give special attention to strengthening the spiritual, emotional, and physical aspects of your flame while fostering forgiveness and self-care, practicing faith, and finding your worthiness. The following seven days, as you're focused on accessing the power of the present, you'll work on igniting freedom, responsibility, humility, acceptance, fearlessness, love, and integrity. And during the final seven days of the cleanse, as you are envisioning your most magnificent self, you'll place your awareness on joy, partnership, and inspiration while nourishing gratitude, passion, compassion, and possibility. By the end of this process, choices that will return you to your truest self will become clearer and easier to make. You'll come to perceive your inner flame and all its nuances as markers letting you know when you are heading in the right direction and when it's time to take a deep breath and release something that is compromising your highest expression. With this new awareness, you will never again feel as though you have lost your way; your gauge will be the strength and force of your glorious internal flame.

In the first stage of the cleanse, you may perceive your inner flame as a mere flicker that is in desperate need of your attention. But as you begin the work of embracing your past and unleashing the power of the present moment, the soft whisper of your soul will begin to gain strength. By the time you nurture all aspects of your internal flame and turn your attention to envisioning a future that inspires and fuels you, the radiance of your roaring fire will light up every room that you enter. Although there will be a few rough days, this process will pull you through, reconnecting you with the divine force that awaits your return.

Each day of the cleanse will bring a new opportunity to rekindle your spirit as you digest the past and bring forth your deepest hopes and desires. As you release old, outworn thoughts, relationships, and strategies, your inner flame will strengthen, and something magical will happen: you'll begin to form a deep and loving relationship with your higher self. As you detoxify your mind and clear away the emotional clutter that drowns out the voice of your heart's true desires, you'll once again be able to hear the call of your own soul. For perhaps the first time since you were a child, you will see clearly enough to discern the path of greatest joy. Each day, rather than being a slave to your ego's insatiable wants and desires, rather than making choices based on what you *think* will bring you happiness and contentment, you will have the ability to listen deeply to the still, small voice that echoes your soul's truth.

The Practice

Each day of the Consciousness Cleanse is designed to be a magical journey into the most mystical aspects of yourself and the universe. Although the cleanse is designed to be done in twenty-one days, if you need a day off or feel a bit overwhelmed by the process, you are welcome to slow down and take a few days to integrate all the insights and wisdom that are being unveiled. You will find that each day is whole unto itself, filled with insights, wisdom, and holy actions that have the power to lift you out of the state of consciousness you are in and into a higher more inspired state of being. There are two essentials you'll need to ensure your success: a new journal in which to share your thoughts and feelings and to record your holy work, and a prayer that soothes your soul or reminds you of the source to which you're returning. If you don't have a

prayer you love, you might consider the beautiful simplicity of
the Serenity Prayer:

> God, grant me the serenity
> To accept the things I cannot change;
> Courage to change the things I can;
> And wisdom to know the difference.

I suggest that each morning you wake up twenty minutes earlier than usual and begin the day by taking some slow, deep
breaths and thanking yourself for embarking on this holy journey. Bless yourself for choosing to reconnect with the divine
force that resides within. Spend some sacred time in prayer,
asking for guidance and strength, and then read over your process work from the previous day. When you feel settled and fully
engaged, you'll begin your morning practice, set your intention
for the day, and create a daily mantra—a sacred phrase that will
nourish and ignite your physical, emotional, and spiritual flames.
This morning practice is simple, short, and potent. Although the
aspects of your flame will change each day in accordance with
the agent of change that you are invoking, the morning practice
will be your grounding cord and will support you in tapping into
the inner wisdom that will serve as your guide and friend.

Please read over the morning practice now and familiarize
yourself with the questions you will be answering. I've also included some examples in order to activate your imagination
and help you to begin to get in touch with the intentions, feelings, and actions that will serve your highest evolution.

You'll begin each morning by taking a few slow, deep breaths and reflecting on the following questions:

- What is the condition of your internal flame right now?

- On a scale of one to ten, where would you rate it? Where would you like it to be at the end of the day?

- What is your intention for the day? What intention can you create to strengthen and fuel your internal flame?

- What is the primary feeling you want to generate from your intention?

- What will you need to do to ensure that your intention becomes a reality?

- What will you have to give up—what thought, belief, or behavior—to ensure that you fulfill your intention for today?

- What healing mantra—what sentence or phrase—can you repeat to yourself throughout the day to soothe your soul and manifest your intention?

- How many times throughout the day do you need to hear this?

If you're focused on nourishing your emotional flame, your morning practice might look something like this:

- My emotional flame feels weak and sad.

- On a scale of one to ten, my flame is a three and I would like it to be a seven by the end of the day.

- My intention for today is to be very kind and compassionate to myself.

- The feeling my intention will generate today is that I am cared for.

- To ensure that my intention becomes a reality, I'll have to forgive myself for being unhappy.

- I will have to give up the thought that my life should be any other way than it is right now.

- My mantra is "I love and accept myself exactly as I am today."

- I need to hear my mantra sixteen times today.

If your daily focus is on strengthening your physical flame, your morning practice might look something like this:

- My physical flame is tired and exhausted.

- On a scale of one to ten, my flame is a six and I would like it to be a nine by the end of the day.

- My intention for today is to love and appreciate my body.

- The feeling my intention will generate today is vitality.

- To ensure that my intention becomes a reality, I'll have to take a nap when my body feels tired.

- I will have to give up the thought that I have no willpower.

- My mantra is "My body is a temple for the divine."

- I need to hear my mantra forty times today.

If your focus for the day is to fuel your spiritual flame, your morning practice might look something like this:

- My spiritual flame feels connected and grateful.

- On a scale of one to ten, my flame is an eight and I would like it to be a ten by the end of the day.

- My intention for today is to feel the presence of God.

- The feeling my intention will generate today is that I am loved.

- To ensure that my intention becomes a reality, I'll have to read a line from a prayer book five times during the day.

- I will have to give up the belief that God isn't paying attention to me.

- My mantra is "I am a beloved child of God."

- I need to hear my mantra seven times today.

If it would help you to hear and experience me guiding you through the morning practice or if you would like to use a daily worksheet, please visit my Web site, debbieford.com/morning-practice, to hear an audio recording of the morning practice or to access worksheets. Once you are clear on your intention—how you want to feel, what you need to do and not do, and what mantra you'll repeat—you'll spend the day dwelling in the distinctions and the questions of that particular day. Even though you might feel compelled to skip the morning practice . . . *don't do it!* You deserve to get everything out of this program and more, so even if you're very excited about getting to the day's reading and cleansing rituals, I recommend that you wait until you are centered and clear about your day's intention before jumping in. The morning practice will ensure that you are open and ready to receive the day's message and indulge in the cleansing rituals.

Next, you'll read the day of the Consciousness Cleanse that applies. Don't worry about doing the exercises first thing in the morning. Just allow the ideas to take root in your awareness, and plan to do your cleansing rituals in the afternoon or when you get home from work. At that time, designate thirty minutes to reading the day again and to answering the questions or doing the cleansing rituals that are prescribed at the end of that day's description.

Every day you will be given a powerful statement to contemplate, to mediate on, and to use to fill your awareness throughout the day. They are designed to remind you, to awaken you, to comfort you, and to begin to encode your consciousness with the very highest resonance. If on any given day you are inspired to select your own source of soul food, please feel free to do so.

At the end of the day, spend a few minutes thanking and acknowledging yourself for taking part in this very deep process. Breathe in and thank God, your soul, and the divine universe that is supporting you in purifying and rejuvenating every aspect of your life. Bring awareness to your breath as you allow the vibration of the powerful statement to return to your awareness and come alive in every cell of your being. Then close your eyes and sleep with the angels.

Cleansing Tools

As you can see, the 21-Day Consciousness Cleanse will deeply support you in making time for the solace of your inner world rather than the busy-ness of your outer world, and therefore it is not a time to conduct "business as usual." Before you begin, it's essential to first create an environment that is safe, nourishing, and uplifting. In this section, I will share some structures and tools that will support you along the way.

FLAME PROTECTORS

- Let the people in your life know that you are taking this time to clear your mind and heart so you can unveil and explore the next stage in the evolution of your soul.

- To the extent that you are able, step away from e-mail, cell phones, television, and other distractions during your cleanse. Record an outgoing phone message letting people know you won't be returning calls until a specified date, or set up an e-mail auto-responder to establish your boundaries during the time you are doing the cleanse.

- Ask the people you interact with on a regular basis to deliver all their communications to you before 6 p.m. on the day before the start of your cleanse, or by a specified time each day, so that you are able to reserve time for yourself and your process.

- Become acutely aware of everything that enters your system—physically, emotionally, and mentally—during the time you are cleansing.

As you prepare for this restorative process, realize that your declaration to bring more divine light into your awareness and more love into your heart may bring up within you everything that stands in the way of your highest good. The Consciousness Cleanse will likely reveal everything that is inconsistent with a pure and high vibration. This is just part of the process—and an important sign, actually, that the process is working. By setting up structures and powerful reminders beforehand, you can use all that arises during the cleanse to your benefit.

Consider putting the following reminders and structures in place to elevate your consciousness while you are in the midst of the cleanse:

CONSCIOUSNESS LIFTERS

- Find several songs that inspire, thrill, and uplift you, and make them into a playlist so you can listen to them often.

- Find a prayer that soothes your soul, and read it each day. (You will find several within the pages of this book.)

- Remember the words of the great Emmet Fox: "If you're thinking about God, you're not thinking about your problems." Surround yourself with sounds, sights, and sensations that remind you of God, love, and an amazing future. If you are present to the possibilities of a life you love, depleting and life-draining thoughts and feelings will be less likely to enter your awareness.

- Move your body every day. Promise yourself that you will release any and all toxicity through movement. Commit to going for daily walks; take a yoga or dance class; or buy a new, inspiring DVD that you can move along with no matter where you are each day. I personally love to do Qigong and find that it's a practice I can maintain even when I am on the road.

- Talk to yourself every day in front of the mirror. Tell yourself in the morning that you—yes, *you*—have the power to move away from anything that is inconsistent with the holiest of vibrations. Affirm to yourself that you are a holy and glorious manifestation of God and that the world needs you. Say this a thousand times a day if you have to.

COMMITMENT BOOSTERS

If your dedication falters and you find yourself saying, "Well, I can just take a day off and go back to my old patterns of thinking and behaving," simply *stop*. Take a long, slow, deep breath, and take a trip into the future . . .

- Journey through time and envision the predictable life that is awaiting you—one that is, in fact, guaranteed—if you don't follow the voice of your soul. Spend an hour visualizing your life exactly as it is now, except that ten years have passed and you're older. This will help to dissolve your resistance and strengthen your resolve.

- If you still feel unwilling to do the work, stand in front of the mirror and repeat this famous phrase: "This isn't cute anymore."

- Make a list of three people you admire and three people you consider to be losers. Then ask yourself, "Which type of person do I want to be?" If you truly desire to actualize your soul's purpose, know that perseverance is the path to that goal.

The Consciousness Cleanse is a golden opportunity to step away from anything that is not of the highest spiritual vibration. No matter how many games we play inside our minds, things aren't going to get better until we pull ourselves out of denial and admit that a great life is not going to happen next week, or next month, or next year—unless we make it happen. Our lives won't get better until we take them on with the same urgency we would use to save a drowning child. Our lives really won't get better until we stop beating ourselves up emotionally and psychologically. There are no seconds to waste. Tomorrow *is* today. Change doesn't happen in the future; it happens right now, by taking action in the present.

The Past

It is the work of a spiritual warrior to tell yourself the truth and to shine a light on the darkness of your past and your inner conflicts. In the next seven days you must bring the love and light of your compassionate heart to the parts of yourself and your life that you have judged harshly, made wrong, or separated from. To reconnect with your true, liberated self, you must look at everything that stands between you and your God-given right to be reunited with your eternal magnificence and ultimately embrace it all.

Although the 21-Day Consciousness Cleanse is a divinely inspired journey to reclaim your light, an essential part of the process is to identify and acknowledge where the war is still being waged within, where there is still darkness. Darkness is nothing more than the absence of light. Darkness looms only where there is toxic buildup and human-made obstacles. Now is your chance to dissolve the past and remove all of your self-imposed limitations—and I mean all of them. This is your opportunity and your challenge to let go of, surrender to, and embrace all that has held you back. It is your opportunity to transform all that has been held in darkness and turn it into light. And the only qualities that you need to bring to this process to ensure your success are willingness, honesty, courage, and compassion.

To prepare yourself to let the light of your soul shine fully, you must first examine where you're internally at war with yourself—where you're giving your power away to the critical voices that wage holy war on your dreams, your hopes, your plans . . . your future. You have to be honest and ask yourself how you repeatedly attack yourself. In this first week you must explore and expose all the ways you withhold the light from your history. How do you participate in creating an inner environment that eases God out? How do you keep yourself lonely, isolated, and disempowered by the limitations of your past? Is it by medicating yourself, by numbing or neglecting yourself, or by depriving yourself of the things that matter most? Is it through listening to demeaning internal dialogue or engaging in damaging and addictive behaviors? You must admit to the choices you make that leave you feeling unsafe and at risk in certain areas of your life or that chisel away at your self-esteem. You must make an honest assessment of your life and see if you are embroiled in an abusive relationship, an unhealthy friendship, or an addiction. In other words, are your dreams and future possibilities held hostage by parts of you that are stuck in the pain of the past?

It is very likely that you've already done a lot of work to transcend the past; please do not let that dishearten you. You may have gathered powerful tools and techniques for personal growth over the years but found that you still bump up against the restrictions of your inner thought process. Whatever your history, I want to assure you that if you have indeed tried and failed, it is only because you were not relying on this powerful force as your guide. In the hands of the ego, techniques and tools can be only so effective. Simply thinking a good thought (i.e., a "spiritually correct" thought) isn't enough. Where people often fall short is in thinking that change, or even transformation, is all about working hard to change the thoughts and beliefs that are embedded in their unconscious mind. This is often a fruitless task. Some of these thoughts and beliefs are passed down from generation to generation. The task of removing them is comparable to trying to excavate the artifacts in a thousand-year-old tomb from beneath five hundred feet of lava—a difficult and life-draining task, unless of course you are being well paid and are contributing to the history of the world by digging them all up, dusting them off, and putting them on view at the public museum of outdated and life-draining beliefs.

You must recognize that there are thousands of life-draining beliefs and if you attach to any of these limiting negative beliefs and call them your own, they become your limitations. So if you can see that being an archaeologist of life-draining beliefs is not your soul's passion or mission, you must let them go.

Beliefs that we make personal become a part of our human ego structure and rob us of experiencing divine realities. As soon as we take them personally, they become our self-imposed limitations. So to melt away the concrete walls that leave our futures "out there," floating somewhere in time, we must come to understand that those things that have blocked us in the first place aren't even ours to claim. They are universal Shadow Beliefs. These beliefs get activated in childhood and adolescence—legacies handed down from our families and society. Until we identify and shine the light of our awareness on these deeply entrenched thought forms and stop taking them personally, they remain as internal roadblocks that sabotage our progress and slow down our forward momentum, no matter how positive our intentions may be. They keep us ego-driven instead of soul-centered. To enter the world of our highest expression, to reconnect with the divine resource that awaits our invitation into utopia, we must step away from the ego's perspective and into the light of divine understanding. If we are truly committed to returning to the expansive radiance of our innocent childlike nature, we must unhook from the beliefs of our past.

This first week of the Consciousness Cleanse will help you to unhook from the limiting and damaging beliefs you've adopted so you can make peace with your past and reclaim your divinity. Each day's process is designed so you can let go of that which is limiting you and cut the cords that bind you to old wounds, hurtful incidents, and undigested loss and heartache. As you disconnect the cords of the ego's control, you will reconnect to your true, authentic nature. Then you will be graced with divine eyes through which life makes sense, and with which you will regain the confidence to be all of who you were meant to be in this lifetime. This heavenly detox will lead you to a place where it is easy to surrender your ego's will to something much greater—a profound and intimate relationship with your soul's passion and eternal power.

When you open up to living inside of the spiritual realm, you're no longer compelled to live according to your outworn beliefs, because you're not referencing your logical mind, your belief system, or your human emotions to tell you where you can go, what you can do, and what's possible for your life. You are referencing the highest truth; you are going to God for your answers and direction. In the realm of divine consciousness, you don't need to know. You also don't need to *not* know. You can see beyond beliefs, beyond knowing, and beyond not knowing. You can allow life to be what it is, and then you can choose to operate on a higher level of consciousness, where you see the good even in the bad, where you see the wisdom in your wounds, where you find the gold in the darkness you've endured. And I can promise you that there is no time better spent for you than that which you spend giving energy, focus, and attention to your divine resource—calling upon it every day to guide, nourish, and sustain you.

In order to become ready to fill your container with the nutrients you need to live a meaningful and purpose-filled existence, you must cleanse. Propelled by this understanding, you will begin the first seven days by becoming clear about your heart's desires and then acknowledging what has worked and is working about life. You will take an honest moral inventory of your behaviors and actions and view yourself and your life from the perspective of an observer.

If you are going to give up the self that you have known yourself to be, it is imperative that you leave your history behind. And to truly do this, it is essential that you milk your past for everything it has to offer—for all the gifts, wisdom, and blessings that it holds. As you begin this sacred process, allow yourself to be present to the fact that you are on a holy journey of living a soul-centered life—a life directed by the greatest force in the universe.

A PRAYER FOR THE PAST

Let all those who guide me support me in peeling away
whatever it is that keeps me blind to what's possible,
that keeps me hidden from my greatness,
that keeps me separate from my loved ones
today I ask you to lighten my heart, to lift my burdens,
my worries, my fears, my anxieties, my grief
so that I may know and cherish all that I am
I see it, I feel it, I acknowledge it right now
and so I know that it is

The Gift of Desire

Desire is the spark that ignites the flame of your soul and illuminates your innate creativity, imagination, and vision. It is the impulse that gives you the ambition and the energy to share your unique talents with the world. Your soul's desires are with you at birth like a hidden treasure chest of possibilities for you to discover as you grow and evolve into the person you were meant to be. Yet before you can harness this powerful force, you must give voice to what you long for in the deepest place in your heart. You may be one of the many who have stopped letting yourself feel the ache of your own desires—either because you are ashamed that some of their desires are self-serving or because you're afraid of the disappointment and hurt you might feel if you don't get what you ask for. But unless you embrace the desires of your heart, you are left empty, estranged from the passion of your soul.

On this day—the first day of this life-altering process—you will summon one of the most powerful agents of change in the universe: *desire*. In its purest form, desire drives you to want something so badly that you are willing to release your outdated behaviors and beliefs in order to manifest it. Desire forces you to grow, evolve, and move closer to your highest expression. Beneath the surface of your ego's insatiable cravings, your authentic desires wait patiently for you to acknowledge and claim them. Gently but persistently they are nudging you to go deeper, to find greater meaning, and to step into a self you have never met before. Desire is your most primal, inborn motivator to become fully expressed, inspired, and passionate and to fulfill your soul's mission on earth. It is one of your most powerful friends and guides.

Today you have the opportunity to unearth the desires that may be covered over with years of fear and resignation—to allow yourself to feel their potency to such a degree that you are willing to fight for their fulfillment. Desire is the most important catalyst for bringing about radical change, so today you're going to reflect on those desires that you most want to bring forth in the next twenty-one days. This is not a dress rehearsal; this is your life. Your time is now. Do not wait another day to become fully engaged in your life, to learn to love and to forgive, and to live with greater purpose and meaning.

CLEANSING RITUALS

- Make a list of all your desires—both those things that you want to achieve in the *outer* world and those that you long to feel *inside*. Do you want more self-confidence, more love, a clearer sense of purpose, greater peace of mind? If so, write it down. Do you desire more money, more friends, a soul mate, a child, or a new career? If so, write it down. This is the time to list all of your desires without censoring yourself. Be honest. Be bold.

- When your list feels complete, separate your desires into "inner" longings and "outer" longings, and then use the following questions to clarify which two desires are most important for you to focus on right now. Ask yourself:

  Why do I want this?

  Is this a desire of my soul?

  What do I hope to experience—internally as well as externally—if I manifest this desire?

  How will the fulfillment of this desire serve the world?

- Now, reflect on your answers and select one inner desire and one outer desire to focus on for the duration of your Consciousness Cleanse. Remember, as you clear away the weeds of doubt, numbness, distraction, sadness, and resignation, you will be better able to nourish the seeds of your desires and bring them to fruition.

- Finally, create a vision map—an outer picture of each of your desires—either by cutting pictures that you love or words that inspire you out of magazines and putting them together in an inspiring way or by adding some images to your screen saver on your computer. Look at your vision map throughout the day to remind yourself of what you truly desire. Commit to taking three minutes each morning to seal these words and images into your consciousness while affirming your Soul Food for the day.

SOUL FOOD
My soul's desire is the voice of God.

MORNING PRACTICE:
IGNITING YOUR SPIRITUAL FLAME

- What is the condition of your spiritual flame right now?

- On a scale of one to ten, where would you rate it? Where would you like it to be at the end of the day?

- What is your intention for the day? What intention can you create to strengthen and fuel your spiritual flame?

- What is the primary feeling you want to generate from your intention?

- What will you need to do to ensure that your intention becomes a reality?

- What will you have to give up—what thought, belief, or behavior—to ensure that you fulfill your intention for today?

- What healing mantra—what sentence or phrase—can you repeat to yourself throughout the day to soothe your soul and manifest your intention?

- How many times throughout the day do you need to hear this?

The Gift of Self-Awareness

Now that you have brought your desires to the surface of your consciousness, it is time to turn your attention to that which is secretly (or maybe not so secretly) robbing you of your soul's desires or standing in your way of fulfilling them. If you are ready to move beyond the repetitive nature of your past, now is the time to become aware of all that has kept you stuck. Take a deep breath. I know the task might seem overwhelming, but I promise you it is not. I've led tens of thousands of people from around the world through the process of unconcealing and embracing their unprocessed shame, guilt, hurt, and remorse, and I know without question that only by releasing the past will you be able to open yourself up to a new, inspiring, and magical future. By reflecting on your past actions from the perspective of an impartial observer, you can distinguish with objectivity the events that are causing you to feel unworthy and unlovable. To aid you in this inquiry, you will enter into a state of reflection where you are able to be aware of your behavior rather than overly identified with it. Unburdened by judgment or biases, you can reflect on your life—past and present—with the clarity that can come only with a large dose of healthy detachment and a commitment to observe yourself from the outside in.

To do this, you must begin to dig deeply into the past and acknowledge the things you wish you had never said or done, and to admit to the choices you've made or failed to make that robbed you of happiness and self-respect. Any behaviors that diminish how you think of yourself or feel inside your body must now be brought into the light of your awareness. If these old behaviors are not purged from the silent recesses of your subconscious, your past resentments, regrets, and judgments will continue to block your connection with the divine source that awaits your return. Until you invoke *self-awareness*—the next agent of change—you will continue to move forward in darkness rather than with the light of awareness. In William Shakespeare's *Twelfth Night*, the Clown declares: "[T]here is no darkness but ignorance." When you fail to bring awareness to the behaviors that have shaped you, you remain ignorant to all that you are and all that you can be. Where there is ignorance, there is intolerance; where there is intolerance, there is darkness; and where there is darkness, there is repetition.

Today, it's time to take a step back and observe from a neutral perspective what you don't like. I will ask you to view your life as though you were watching a movie or television show, looking—with a bit of distance—to see what you like and don't like about your life and what turns you off and robs you of your energy. What is called for now is to take an inventory of your behaviors with the same degree of detachment you would feel if you walked into a Target store and started counting lawn mowers on the shelves. This kind of clear-eyed, neutral evaluation and accounting requires a commitment to see the truth about yourself and your actions without berating or shaming yourself. Chances are high that there has been enough of that already, and it has never resulted in any positive, forward movement. Today you have an opportunity to bring a refreshing level of honesty and sobriety to the process of reflecting on your behavior. The act of honest, unprejudiced reflection will allow the light of awareness to enter your consciousness.

CLEANSING RITUALS

Today is the day to take an honest inventory—a "searching and fearless" inventory, as they say in the 12-Step process, and not a bitter and blaming one—of all the undigested experiences that are still creating toxicity within your mind and body. Approach this process with vigor, knowing that it is an essential step in preparing your consciousness for the glorious things to come.

- Find a quiet place where you will not be interrupted, and take out your journal. Reflect on each of the following questions, allowing yourself to freely express anything that comes up, without censoring or judging yourself:

  What do I wish I had never done?

  What do I wish I could forget?

  What do I wish I could do differently?

  What behaviors have I participated in that intentionally or unintentionally brought harm to others?

  If you find this journaling exercise degenerating into the retelling of a negative story about you or your life, you must catch yourself. Stop, take a breath, and step outside the story and back into the neutral zone of awareness. If you find yourself sinking into emotions like sadness, regret, anger, or resentment, just gently remind yourself that you're taking this process too personally, and use your breath to help move yourself along.

- Make a list of everything that has ever gone wrong in your life that you have taken too personally.

- How have you punished yourself? What do you do to beat yourself up?

- What are all the reasons you believe you hold on to them?

Once you feel complete with your inventory, you may wonder what you need to do about everything you have written. The answer is: nothing. Nothing at all. For now, I ask that you trust the process; I ask you to trust that the act of digging deeply and getting this inner residue outside of you and onto the pages of your journal will have a transformative power all its own.

- Now, take another deep breath and write down what would be available to you if you allowed all of your human behaviors, thoughts, feelings, and experiences to live outside of yourself—one arm's length away from you—from now on.

SOUL FOOD
My darkness is an absence of light.

MORNING PRACTICE:
IGNITING YOUR EMOTIONAL FLAME

- What is the condition of your emotional flame right now?

- On a scale of one to ten, where would you rate it? Where would you like it to be at the end of the day?

- What is your intention for the day? What intention can you create to strengthen and fuel your emotional flame?

- What is the primary feeling you want to generate from your intention?

- What will you need to do to ensure that your intention becomes a reality?

- What will you have to give up—what thought, belief, or behavior—to ensure that you fulfill your intention for today?

- What healing mantra—what sentence or phrase—can you repeat to yourself throughout the day to soothe your soul and manifest your intention?

- How many times throughout the day do you need to hear this?

The Gift of Release

To keep the vessel of your consciousness cleansed, you have to release what accumulates within it. There is a pure state of being that comes easy to you when you're young, before you encounter people and experiences that shame you, wound you, and douse your internal flame. So to move deeper into the Consciousness Cleanse, you must invoke today's agent of change called *release* as you seek out and let go of what has robbed you of the purity of an innocent mind, a clear heart, and a strong body.

All transformation begins when you can see your life and experiences through new eyes. When you revisit your past, it is literally as if you are exploring a cellar that hasn't been entered or cleaned out in years. When you are courageous enough to step in, armed with this most powerful agent of change, you take on the task with calm and certainty. Most people try to clean out their basements alone, and they wind up feeling too scared or too overwhelmed by the stench and enormity of what's rotten, old, or dead. So after just a few minutes or hours they turn around, walk back up the stairs, and lock the door behind them. Then, no matter how hard they try to convince themselves that there isn't a dirty, filthy cellar locked inside their consciousness, in times of stress it will be exposed.

Imagine that for every negative thing that's ever been said or done to you, a little pellet of pesticide has entered your bloodstream. Allow yourself to reflect on all the years and all the people who have impacted you in a negative way. All the people who said:

> *You didn't do that right.*
> *You made a mistake.*
> *You should be kinder.*
> *You're so stupid.*
> *No one will ever love you.*
> *You can't do anything right.*
> *You're just too needy.*
> *You're a little overweight for my taste.*
> *You're angry.*
> *You're a selfish bitch.*
> *All you ever do is think about yourself.*

Imagine all those words as poisonous black beads being dropped into your awareness. How much toxicity do you think has built up inside your consciousness as a result of your internalization of those kinds of words alone?

And now think about the things you have said to yourself, the anxieties and insecurities you've obsessed over, the fearful judgments you have believed to be true:

I'm not good enough, smart enough, educated enough, pretty enough, talented enough . . .
I'm not as good as . . .

Imagine all the damaging things you've said to yourself as little drops of pesticide that have entered your consciousness, blocking your ability to see the fullness of your magnificence and your divinity. How many of these poisonous pellets are there? How thick and sticky are they? What are they doing to your connection to spirit?

Now that you are aware of this inner toxicity, imagine it taking form. What size is it? What color is it? In pounds, how much does it weigh? What effect does it have on your body? Can you see that you have locked away a ton of toxic mold in the cellar of your precious psyche? Now that you've begun to expose the clutter and stench of your inner chambers by engaging in this inquiry, it's time to open the door and begin the holy process of releasing it all and letting God sweep out your cellar and haul away the toxic mold of the past. When you are complete, you will feel so pure inside that you'll be happy to revisit your beautiful basement anytime.

CLEANSING RITUALS

- Take some time to reflect on what has interrupted and corrupted your pure and natural state. What is, right here and now, acting like a toxic spill within the pristine environment of your conscious heart?

- Allow yourself to see how this toxicity has hurt you. On a scale from one to ten, with one being "not much" and ten being "more than you can calculate," rate how this buildup of emotional and mental toxicity has blocked your flow of well-being and has stolen vitality from you in the following core areas. (Circle one number for each item.)

My self-esteem	1–2–3–4–5–6–7–8–9–10
My confidence	1–2–3–4–5–6–7–8–9–10
My physical energy	1–2–3–4–5–6–7–8–9–10
My creativity	1–2–3–4–5–6–7–8–9–10
My passion	1–2–3–4–5–6–7–8–9–10
My intuition	1–2–3–4–5–6–7–8–9–10
My future	1–2–3–4–5–6–7–8–9–10
My sense of peace	1–2–3–4–5–6–7–8–9–10

My ability to love   1–2–3–4–5–6–7–8–9–10

My ability to be loved   1–2–3–4–5–6–7–8–9–10

- Remembering that the truth will set you free, take this journaling time to admit to what is still poisoning your consciousness at this point in your life. What is lurking around in your psyche that is negatively affecting your ability to have more love, joy, happiness, and success?

- Take the time to draw a picture of what's been hidden inside your psyche. What size, shape, color, and weight is it? As you draw, allow yourself to feel the release of getting it off your chest, off your back, off your mind, and out of your body. Remember, if you can externalize the accumulation of toxicity, you won't need to internalize it.

- When you are done, place your drawing in a steel bowl or fire pit, set it on fire, and watch the toxicity of the past turn to ash as you chant the following words silently or aloud:

    I give this to you, God, to transform into nectar for my soul. I let go of all that has taken up space in my mind, body, and psyche. I give to you all the pain that I've been unable to let go of. Today, I ask that you turn what has formerly been toxic into fuel for my future.

- Now, write a short story about your life free from the toxicity of your past. Allow yourself to dream an easy, carefree future filled with fun and frolic. Be creative as you describe your walk, your sense of well-being, and your deep gratitude for life. Give yourself the gift today of dreaming a new future.

SOUL FOOD
I am released from the bondage of my past.

MORNING PRACTICE:
IGNITING YOUR PHYSICAL FLAME

- What is the condition of your physical flame right now?

- On a scale of one to ten, where would you rate it? Where would you like it to be at the end of the day?

- What is your intention for the day? What intention can you create to strengthen and fuel your physical flame?

- What is the primary feeling you want to generate from your intention?

- What will you need to do to ensure that your intention becomes a reality?

- What will you have to give up—what thought, belief, or behavior—to ensure that you fulfill your intention for today?

- What healing mantra—what sentence or phrase—can you repeat to yourself throughout the day to soothe your soul and manifest your intention?

- How many times throughout the day do you need to hear this?

The Gift of Forgiveness

You have to pray to be released from the toxic poison of your mind so that you may be free to transcend the limitations of your past. You must give up all your old ways of thinking, being, acting, and behaving in order to form new patterns of life based on who you know you can be rather than who you've been in your past. And you cannot do this until you release your ties to those who have harmed you, left you, deceived you, or hurt you in any other way.

As you open up to higher realms of love, peace, and joy, you see that the ticket into these levels of reality is *forgiveness*—your next agent of change. Without forgiving all those you have harbored bad feelings toward, you continue to be imprisoned by your past. If you do not cut the cords of resentment, you will be held captive by the very people you are trying to get away from. Without activating this most powerful agent of change, you will continually have hooks binding you to the incidents that caused the resentment in the first place. Because the outer world is a reflection of your inner world, these hooks throw out energy and will ensure that you re-create, in other situations, the same bad feelings you are holding on to inside yourself. Who wants to do that? It's bad enough that you have been hurt so deeply that you still remember the event for days, weeks, years, or decades, but then the kicker is that your grudges become your jailers, locking you into thought patterns, habits, and feelings that deny you your soul's expression.

Unknowingly, your resentments define who you are and who you can be in the future, because you can be only as great as the size of your heart. And if your ability to love from deep in your heart is clouded by the experiences of the past, you are in a lose-lose situation. You first lose your freedom when something penetrates your emotional body and affects you so painfully. And you lose again when you decide to hold on to the bad feelings instead of turning them into powerful fuel for the future.

Resentments and grudges are the culprits that cause you to remain in the cycles of self-abuse, negativity, and victimhood. They lodge inside you, causing you to lose touch with your inherent worth, your joy, and—more important—your God-loving heart. To live in the present moment and open yourself to every new great experience to come, you must forgive the past and leave it where it belongs—in the past. Today you have to fight for your freedom just as so many before you have done. The fight now is not so much with your outer restrictions, although there are many, but with the inner confines that keep you trapped in the ugly, barren prison of your mind and your heart. As you say good-bye to the grief, resentments, and disappointments that shape your thoughts, that create your feelings, that cause you to react instead of act, to fight instead of surrender, to shut down instead of open up, to push away rather than allow in, and to judge instead of love—as you say good-bye to all this, you will discover that every person, situation, and painful incident comes bearing gifts. The gifts are often hidden from you until you take the courageous step into forgiveness. Although I don't believe that it is a process you can engage in at will, you can begin invoking this heart-healing agent of change by asking God to be your guide and your supporter. You can ask the powers that be to show you the gifts that you may mine from the darkness of your hurt heart. You can ask God to give you access to a larger perspective so you can see why you chose to go through what you went through in this lifetime.

CLEANSING RITUALS

- Identify the grudges, resentments, and disappointments you have been carrying around with you.

- Calculate how long you have been holding on to those grudges and resentments—how many minutes, hours, days, months, years, or decades.

- Identify the cost of holding on to them. Does it cost you energy, vitality, self-esteem, intimacy?

- Tracing your grudges back to specific incidents and experiences, identify how you took personally the hurt these incidents caused you.

- If these experiences were designed to deliver you some wisdom or some gift, what would that be?

- Allow yourself to see what would become available to you if you allowed God to take your grudges from you. What could open up in your life that isn't open to you right now?

- Write a letter expressing your feelings and asking God to release you from the prison of your resentments, grudges, and disappointments.

SOUL FOOD
Forgive me for my trespasses as I forgive those who trespass against me.

MORNING PRACTICE:
IGNITING YOUR FORGIVENESS FLAME

- What is the condition of your forgiveness flame right now?

- On a scale of one to ten, where would you rate it? Where would you like it to be at the end of the day?

- What is your intention for the day? What intention can you create to strengthen and fuel your forgiveness flame?

- What is the primary feeling you want to generate from your intention?

- What will you need to do to ensure that your intention becomes a reality?

- What will you have to give up—what thought, belief, or behavior—to ensure that you fulfill your intention for today?

- What healing mantra—what sentence or phrase—can you repeat to yourself throughout the day to soothe your soul and manifest your intention?

- How many times throughout the day do you need to hear this?

The Gift of Reverence

Your body is your temple. It is the home of the Divine, the resting place of the holy. Without it, you cannot express the glory of the Divine on this earth. Even though you are not your body—you are simply using it as a vessel to play this game of human life—your body is a sacred container on loan to you for a very short while.

You might think you would be humbled and honored to be handed a playing piece so valuable that it permits you access to the game of life. You might believe you are a kind and appreciative person who, if given the opportunity to inhabit the earth and manifest a unique expression of God, would remain grateful and treat your body like the divine gift that it is. One would think that since the only "buy-in" to the game was this body of yours, you would hold it, nourish it, adore it, and revere it each day that you were blessed to embody it. But this might not be the case. Maybe your body shows up like a nuisance, another thing that has to be fed, cared for, and maintained—another to-do on your long list of tasks that must be checked off.

My friend Cheryl Richardson, author of *The Art of Extreme Self-Care*, always reminds me that "the foundation of a good life is good health." To transform your relationship with your body, you must embrace the agent of change known as *reverence*. When you are present to the absolute gift that you have been blessed with—the sacredness of having a body—you will begin to move in the world with more grace, gratitude, and humility than you ever thought possible. You naturally become more sensitive to your own needs and focus on caring for yourself in a kinder, gentler way. When you guard your body each day as if it were a million pounds of gold and treat yourself with the respect and kindness that you would give to one of your favorite spiritual heroes, your body becomes the doorway to new levels of self-love and spiritual fuel. The facts are these: The more love and reverence you give your body, the better you will feel. The more attention you give your sacred container, the more divine power it will be able to hold.

To step into reverence for your body, you must forgive yourself for all you have done and not done to care for it. You must bless what is good about your beautiful body and find acceptance for all you have deemed to be wrong or bad. You must be present to all that it does each day to keep you alive and in the game of life. And bless it for the opportunity it gives you to evolve your soul. Bless your body, and it will bless you back. This is your sacred task today.

CLEANSING RITUALS

The next step in purifying your consciousness is to make the commitment to treat your body with reverence.

- Make a list of the ways you've given your energy away, abused yourself, ignored your needs, stepped over your boundaries, and given more than you had to give. Freely express all the times you have hated your body for getting sick or run down. Acknowledge the ways you've ignored the messages your body was sending you. Add to the list all the times you've chosen to engage in an activity when you were exhausted; all the ways you've criticized your body for being too short, fat, slow, or different; all the times you've been insensitive to the care that your body needs.

- As you read over this list, allow yourself to say "I'm sorry" to the sacred vessel that exists for the sole purpose of allowing you to express your divine gifts. This is the time to apologize for all the times you didn't rest, when you put somebody else's needs above your own, or exercised too hard, or when you chose foods or drugs that were emotional Band-Aids rather than what your body needed to replenish itself and gain energy.

- Today, write a letter to your body asking for forgiveness. Your letter might look something like this: "I'm sorry for hating myself: for being too skinny or fat, short or tall. I'm sorry for eating cupcakes when my body needed grains. For not taking the time to stretch before my workout." If you knew that your body was the holy container of the Divine, what do you need to say you're sorry for?

- Your body has the ability to tell you what it needs to be healthy and vital, but to hear its messages, you must become sensitive to it. Your body needs to be exercised, to be cared for, nourished, and replenished. It needs sunshine, good food, rest, nutrients, stretching, and care in the form of a dentist or a doctor. This is the day to become sensitive to the needs of your body. If you need to have a checkup or take care of some part of your body, make the appointment today.

- Now take a few minutes to read over this prayer for healing and energy. Allow these words to penetrate your consciousness.

I allow myself to feel the endless energy of the Universe

I drink from the river of pure potentiality

I sip the sweet drops of life force

So that they can fill my body with vitality

I feel the endless energy of my youth filling my body,

enlivening my spirit, restoring me to perfect health

Wholeness and happiness are my birthright

My constant companions

Appreciation for my body medicine for my soul

SOUL FOOD
I revere my body as a sacred container of God.

MORNING PRACTICE:
IGNITING YOUR SELF-CARE FLAME

- What is the condition of your self-care flame right now?

- On a scale of one to ten, where would you rate it? Where would you like it to be at the end of the day?

- What is your intention for the day? What intention can you create to strengthen and fuel your self-care flame?

- What is the primary feeling you want to generate from your intention?

- What will you need to do to ensure that your intention becomes a reality?

- What will you have to give up—what thought, belief, or behavior—to ensure that you fulfill your intention for today?

- What healing mantra—what sentence or phrase—can you repeat to yourself throughout the day to soothe your soul and manifest your intention?

- How many times throughout the day do you need to hear this?

The Gift of Surrender

Today, you may be more aware of some of your feelings. Uncomfortable emotions may be emerging within you, signaling that feelings you've long suppressed are now coming to the surface. It's vital to this process that you take a deep breath and allow them in. Invite your turbulent memories, and the unwelcome emotions they carry with them, to surface, trusting that the only way out is through. Give yourself permission to feel whatever is happening within your body without expending any of your precious energy trying to manage, hide, or deny your experience. This is not a time to eat, drink, gossip, or shop in order to numb what you are feeling inside. It's a sacred time, an opportunity to listen intently to that which you have routinely disavowed. To facilitate this healing process, today you can engage the agent of change known as *surrender*. Breathe that in. You are about to *allow* your feelings to exist by surrendering them to a power greater than yourself.

When you allow your emotions to be as they are—without trying to fix, change, or deny them—something magical happens: they pass through you. But when you resist your emotions, when you invest your energy in wishing and wanting to feel different than you do, you have to find ways to indulge yourself in quick fixes, giving up your soulful dreams for short-lived gratification. When you are wishing away your feelings of loss, hurt, anger, or loneliness and wanting to feel different than you do, you block the natural outlets that enable your emotions to move through you. Your feelings are meant to inform you when your needs are not being met. Suppressing them not only deprives you of their wisdom, but results in an accumulation of resistance that obstructs your connection to your divine resource.

It's important to understand that you resist your feelings only when you take them personally or when you believe that experiencing certain feelings means something about who you are—about your character, your value, or your acceptability to others. You withhold and suppress your emotions when you believe that expressing your feelings might actually jeopardize your place of belonging in the world. If you feel angry, you might tell yourself that something is wrong with you or that you are mean. If you feel scared, you may interpret it as evidence that you are unlovable, incompetent, unworthy, or incapable of taking care of yourself. It's your interpretations of your emotions—not the emotions themselves—that you resist the most.

You must have faith that your feelings exist to inform you. They are often your soul's way to communicate to you. If you deny them, suppress them by overeating, or pretend they are not real, they can't help you in finding your way back home and into the arms of the Divine. Your difficult feelings need love, too. And people who ignore them long enough will be left in a state of deep depression and/or resignation. If someone leaves you, it's normal for you to feel sad. When granted the right to exist, your sadness can become a healing balm, an actual psychic release that is meant to clear away and release human experiences. No doubt you have experienced the relief that comes after a much-needed cry; there's nothing like it. But when you resist what you feel, your sadness, compounded with your harsh judgments, affects your lovability and self-esteem. You bind yourself in an endless loop of hopelessness and despair . . . and for far too long. By granting your feelings the right to exist, you melt away these interpretations layer by layer and cleanse the lens through which you see yourself and the world. By surrendering your feelings into the arms of your higher power, you join forces with the Divine, and toxic emotions can be transformed into evolutionary food for your soul.

Today I will ask you to bring the same compassion and loving-kindness to your own sweet self that you would extend to a child or to a loved one in need. I ask you to breathe into whatever feelings you are experiencing right now, without giving in to the habit of trying to fix, change, or suppress them. Today is a day to have faith and create a relaxing environment of permission, tolerance, and spaciousness within yourself. With the grace with which a tender lover might take you in their arms, surrendering to what is real for you in this moment welcomes and embraces all your human emotions.

CLEANSING RITUALS

Today, I invite you to experiment with a simple process that can bring a sense of relief and peace into your consciousness.

- Make a list of all the feelings you have deemed wrong, awful, scary, or otherwise unacceptable. Include feelings you have experienced as well as those you never want to experience. Remember, today's agent of change asks you for nothing less than to surrender all of your feelings to a higher power. You begin to do so by allowing whatever comes up to be there, so don't hold back. After you've made your list, identify the *top three* emotions that you resist the most.

- Reflect on each of these feelings and notice what comes into your awareness as you ask the following questions:

  How old was I when I deemed them wrong or unacceptable?

How have I resisted these emotions?

How do I try to manage or control these feelings?

What behaviors have I used to avoid, ignore, and deny their existence?

- Ask your higher self to show you how these feelings could serve you in the future if you just allowed them to be.

What gifts have these emotions brought me?

What lessons have I learned by either expressing them or resisting them?

What wisdom do they hold for me?

What would be available to me if I simply allowed these feelings to exist exactly as they are? Would I experience more peace? More freedom? More ease?

Notice what happens when you choose to embrace rather than reject each feeling that arises within you today. This process of allowing yourself to just feel your feelings can bring miraculous and unexpected opportunities, internally and externally.

SOUL FOOD
Divine goodness awaits me.

MORNING PRACTICE:
IGNITING YOUR FAITH FLAME

- What is the condition of your faith flame right now?

- On a scale of one to ten, where would you rate it? Where would you like it to be at the end of the day?

- What is your intention for the day? What intention can you create to strengthen and fuel your faith flame?

- What is the primary feeling you want to generate from your intention?

- What will you need to do to ensure that your intention becomes a reality?

- What will you have to give up—what thought, belief, or behavior—to ensure that you fulfill your intention for today?

- What healing mantra—what sentence or phrase—can you repeat to yourself throughout the day to soothe your soul and manifest your intention?

- How many times throughout the day do you need to hear this?

The Gift of Self-Acknowledgment

The sacred process of self-acknowledgment is the act of consciously and deliberately celebrating the best in yourself. In the presence of your own loving attention, you create the inner conditions that are necessary to step into the next greatest evolution of yourself. Right now, there is a stronger, more vibrant, more inspired version of "you" that is wanting and waiting to emerge. Because you are a living, growing being, your consciousness will continue to evolve, and your expression will continue to expand. Take a moment to consider what this means for you personally . . . *the next greatest evolution of yourself.*

By embracing *self-acknowledgment*—today's potent agent of change—you will take the next step in clearing out and opening up your consciousness to receive the peace, joy, and fulfillment you are seeking. Self-acknowledgment boosts your emotional and spiritual immunity, giving you the perspective you need to release the past and rise above resignation and hopelessness. By affirming your own gifts and strengths, you build your confidence and increase your ability to build a brighter future.

Today you will deliberately turn your attention to all that you have done well in the past, to all that you value and appreciate about yourself, to the courageous actions you've taken, to the things you've accomplished, and to the contributions you've made to the people around you. Today is the day to focus 100 percent of your attention on what you love about yourself and on all that is going well in your life. Self-acknowledgment is truly a holy practice.

CLEANSING RITUALS

- You start this milestone day by taking an inventory of all that you want to be acknowledged for. Beginning with the first ten years of your life, make a list of all the things you deserve to be acknowledged for, and continue this process decade by decade until you arrive at your current age. If you can take a bit more time as you reflect on the last two years of your life, list your acknowledgments month by month. If you get stuck, ask your friends and family members to tell you what they love most about you and what they will remember about you when you die. If the things they share ring true and light you up, add them to your list.

- Now take some time to take in the depth and breadth of your list. Remember, this is the beginning of a process that will change the way you see yourself and therefore alter the way you see the world. Read—aloud, if possible—the first thing on your list. Breathe this statement of acknowledgment into your body, affirming that you indeed did take this action, deliver this gift, attain this goal, or contribute in this way. Then close your eyes and repeat the acknowledgment, breathing the words into every cell of your body and allowing the sound of your own voice to serve as an anchor for the significance of these achievements. As you acknowledge each positive action and behavior, allow yourself to relax more and more and to sink into the divine space of seeing and feeling your own greatness.

I invite you to take this process on as if you were writing the list for a ten-year-old child who will use it to gather some of their self-esteem. When were you strong? When did you help someone out? When did you stand up for yourself or another? When did you defy the odds and achieve something you wanted? When did you take a risk that worked out? When did you find the courage to apologize for something you were sorry for? What qualities are used to describe you that you are most proud of? Be very generous with yourself throughout this process.

I know this might seem a giant undertaking for one day—and this is intentional. You should be so busy today thinking about all your successes, your gifts, your contributions, and your positive aspects that you have no time to think about anything else. And please enjoy today: it is a celebration of your soul's journey thus far.

SOUL FOOD
My worth is celebrated by all.

MORNING PRACTICE:
IGNITING YOUR WORTHINESS FLAME

- What is the condition of your worthiness flame right now?

- On a scale of one to ten, where would you rate it? Where would you like it to be at the end of the day?

- What is your intention for the day? What intention can you create to strengthen and fuel your worthiness flame?

- What is the primary feeling you want to generate from your intention?

- What will you need to do to ensure that your intention becomes a reality?

- What will you have to give up—what thought, belief, or behavior—to ensure that you fulfill your intention for today?

- What healing mantra—what sentence or phrase—can you repeat to yourself throughout the day to soothe your soul and manifest your intention?

- How many times throughout the day do you need to hear this?

The Present

As you prepare to enter the second week of the Consciousness Cleanse, I invite you to acknowledge how deeply you have traveled during week one. You did it. You have already given yourself the gift of seven illuminating days of self-observation and self-inquiry. You're well on your way to unhooking from the outer world in order to heed the sweet call of your soul, the voice that is calling you toward an extraordinary future. You have also unconcealed and examined many of the beliefs and behaviors that have hindered you, resulting in too many letdowns and too much suffering in your life. But here is one of the core truths that I want you to claim for yourself as you begin this next phase of the process: *all suffering is rooted in misperception.*

Maybe you believe that life should be better than it is this day. You may believe that you should be more, better, and different than the way you are, and you probably expect others to be more, better, and different than they are. This mind-set causes you to often be dissatisfied. It causes you to get on the proverbial treadmill and chase one more thing in the outer world that promises to give you inner satisfaction. But it is a cosmic joke, a twisted paradox—because if you really do find something to fill the hole for a while, you will be seduced into believing that you can fill the hole from the outside in. Then you are sucked in, for what seems like an eternity, to trying to find the next quick fix to satisfy the hole in your soul. On the other hand, if you do not find the thing to fill the hole, you are tricked into believing that you will be satisfied the moment you do find that one thing out there that will fill it for a while. So in a sense, you are screwed either way. You are damned if you do, and doomed if you do not, to living a life of wanting and waiting for the great fulfillment to come your way.

This is why we must all *stop*, take a breather, cleanse our consciousness of these misperceptions, and remind ourselves that this outer journey is really an inner calling. The call is to return home to the limitless, expansive pool of divine oneness, which is the only spiritual food that will satisfy the eternal emptiness that plagues our human existence. Until we open our eyes to what lies beneath the surface of the self that we know, we will have to continue the exhausting chase for more, better, and different than what we already have. The chase won't end until we find and reclaim our golden essence and allow ourselves to step into the gigantic expression of our soul's unique journey. Until then, we will have to try to fit into a life that is too small, too confining, and too limiting for our soul's fulfillment. We will have to continue to believe that we are small, individual beings rather than a piece of a gigantic collective heart and a molecule of the divine power. We will have to continue to follow the human ego's arduous journey to outer fulfillment, with all of the painful constrictions that this entails. This is the root of our suffering: trying to squeeze ourselves into a shoe that doesn't fit, one that is way too small for our eternal essence.

I once heard an old Sufi story that illustrates with simple clarity how the human self insists on wearing garments that are sometimes too small and tight to give us the comfort we're seeking.

A woman says to her friend, "Poor Lila really has suffered for what she believes."

Her friend asks, "What *does* Lila believe in?"

"Lila believes that she can continue to wear a size six pair of shoes on her size nine feet."

"How painful," her friend murmurs. "What can we do to help?"

"We cannot do a thing except pray that the ill-fitting shoes come apart at the seams and Lila is forced to finally throw them away."

Lila walks around, day after day, pinching off her power—

forcing herself into limping through life as a diminished version of who she was born to be. This tendency presents one of the big challenges for us human beings—to stop tolerating mediocrity and trying to stay small when the truth is that we are capable of great things. We frequently hide our true greatness by staying in jobs, relationships, friendships, and habits that dim our light and diminish out spirit. The pressure and grief that we experience when we are trying to stay within the parameters of a self that is smaller than our soul's contribution is a suffering that most of us cannot bear.

If you are willing, just close your eyes for a moment and call forth the voice of the highest power in the universe. Take a deep breath, and ask, "Where am I suffering right now?" When you get your answer, just breathe in, thank the part of you that is willing to admit to this truth, and allow yourself to become aware of all the ways that you keep trying to squeeze your foot into a shoe that is too small—a life that falls short of your soul's potential.

Now, why would you tolerate the pain of a constricting old identity—why would you tolerate this oppressive pinch when the truth of who you are is so much greater? The reason you squeeze yourself into shoes that are clearly too small is because you have lost your faith to one degree or another. You have lost faith either in yourself, in those whom you share the planet with, in the presence of a divine source, or the possibility of a future filled with love, passion, and endless possibilities.

If you look, you will find an aspect of yourself that is faithless—the part of you that has fallen to its knees, knocked down by heartbreak and stripped of faith after years of disappointments and difficulties of all kinds. Pummeled and bruised by the painful moments in life, this faithless part of you clings stubbornly and desperately to what it knows. Lost and alone, this part of you keeps forcing the size-six shoes onto your size-nine feet. Never mind that these shoes have holes in the bottom and their sparkling sheen is long gone. Forget about the fact that you can barely stand upright in them. Your faithless self holds on anyway, because at least that part of you *knows* those shoes. At least the discomfort they inflict is *predictable*. But with a bit of scrutiny, you can see the paradox: your faithless self actually does have its own brand of faith. It's a kind of misplaced faith—faith in your limitations, faith in your blockages, faith in your negative internal dialogue.

OK, but now that you can see beyond your past, beyond your outdated beliefs, assumptions, and habitual patterns, you can say, "Enough is enough." You can declare the eighth day of the Consciousness Cleanse to be a demarcation, etched in stone, of the turning of the tide. Today you can make a commitment that you will *no longer* put up with needless suffering, emotional pain, and the repetitive bad habits of your past. Your arrival at week two of the cleanse is evidence of that fact. The force with which your soul is calling you toward your deeper purpose will never settle for faux faith. It wants the real thing. And so the seven days you're about to enter into are an opportunity to take your faith-less self gently by the hand, letting it know that you understand its trepidation but that you also know that everything it really wants requires that it kick off the shoes of the past. Simply let it know that you're partnering with it. You and your faithless self are taking one step at a time together into your larger shoes, the ones that your own soul has had tailor-made for you. And to-gether you can stand firmly—and comfortably—in the power of your present.

Today is the day when you move into the present moment, the day when you shift from living a past-driven experience to one of divine creation. And so it is in that spirit of creation that I want you to answer the following questions:

> Are you willing, for the next fourteen days of the cleanse, to let go of any self-criticism or negative internal dialogue that you are still holding?
>
> Are you willing to join forces with your divine self to further cleanse your consciousness and plant new, holy, fertile seeds?

This is not an easy task, but it is the only one worthy of committing your life to each day. So please step forward in faith. Reach out your hand, and ask God to lead you closer to the light. Trust that you are on the right path, entering a new day—a new level of consciousness where the only thing that matters is being rooted in and filled up with the love, light, and compassion of the greatest power in the universe.

A PRAYER FOR THE PRESENT

Creator of the universe,
bless me on this day to make this moment holy
bring forth in me the light so that
I may know myself in the deepest way, in every way
help me keep my heart open and humble
allow me the gracious gift of the precious present
so that I can bring joy and comfort
to all that I love
I see it, I feel it, I acknowledge it right now
and so I know that it is

The Power of Liberation

As you move out of the past and open up to the present, you wake up into a new day, a new time, where you are free to be all you ever imagined. The weight you have carried for far too long gets dropped. Like Grasper, you molt and step into the realm that Deepak Chopra would call the field of infinite possibilities—the field of consciousness where you are one with all that is, all that was, and all that will be; the field where you see with clear and open eyes and are infused with the certainty that you can live a life that truly matters.

But before you go there, you want to ensure that you're really leaving the past where it's meant to be . . . *in the past.* So today will be a rite of passage—a day of celebration and ceremony where you will invoke the next agent of change, called *liberation*, and release all that reminds you of the past, everything that is symbolic of your pain, your anger, and your attachment to old ways of being. Today, in your first step forward into the present, you can joyously be like a child who is making the transition from boy to man or from girl to woman as you offer up your past to a power greater than yourself. Yes, you are summoning the courage to kick off the small shoes of the past that you've stuffed your tender and aching feet into for too many miles, too many years.

CLEANSING RITUALS

Preparation for the Ceremony

- Tonight, you're going to perform a ceremony in which you energetically let go of your physical and emotional past. You're going to dust it off, pray it off, dance it off, sing it off, wash it off, and send it off. In preparation, gather whatever symbols remind you of the limitations of the past. Think about the shoes. In fact, you might own a pair that have literally been squeezing your feet, breaking your back, and hampering the full expression of your feet, so to speak. You might have old journals, pictures that bring up bad feelings, clothes that no longer fit or are symbolic of a "you" that you no longer care to express. Maybe you've been trapped inside an addiction to some food—say, cookies, cupcakes, or salted pretzels. Get a few for the ceremony.

- Next, you're going to write a letter saying good-bye to all the people, places, and things that no longer serve you—the addictions, habits, thoughts, beliefs, feelings, stories, dramas, traumas, and anything else you can think of that fits into this category called "the past you're ready to leave behind."

- You're going to declare today as a demarcation point, a day that you will remember for the rest of your life, one on which you deeply acknowledge the enormity of what you've gone through in your life. This is a day of celebration, so no matter what you're doing—working from home, going to the office, doing something with your kids—you'll want to dress up as if it's one of the most important days of your life. Symbolically, this is a wedding day on which you marry into the present moment, where you choose God as your partner and "doing it alone" becomes an option of the past. Take the time today to buy yourself some flowers, pick up a scented candle, or download some special music, so that all of your attention this evening can be focused on what you're going to leave behind.

- Take today as a day to *not* turn on your TV, look at your computer, or worry about returning your phone calls.

Instead, claim it as your day to take time away from life in order to fully enjoy this holy passage. And remember to ask the powers that be to join you in this sacred process.

- With your candles, flowers, music, incense, and anything else you've chosen to set the tone, create a special environment for your sacred ceremony. Select a place where you can be alone and uninterrupted for an hour. This needs to be a place where you are free to speak out loud, because the power of your own spoken words will resonate through every cell, through every bit of consciousness that you hold.

- Since you can release only what you bless, bring all the things you gathered up earlier that you're now ready to throw away—the letters, photos, clothes, shoes, and more. And if possible, use your home computer and printer to generate signs saying "THE PAST" that you can tape to each item you're releasing or to the container you're releasing them into.

- For the more intangibles: on little pieces of paper, write down the beliefs and behaviors that have limited you— for example, "This is my addiction to the news"; "This is my belief that I'm not good enough"; "This is my belief that I'm too old." Maybe you've been holding on to a nasty note or an old e-mail that somebody sent you or a picture with someone who now reflects a sour memory. This is the time to let them all go.

- I know you may not be able to make a bonfire or have a safe place to burn anything, so get yourself a nice black garbage bag instead. It will serve as your ceremonial container for discarding the tokens of the past.

THE CEREMONY

- Pick up your first item. Is it a piece of paper or a letter that's carrying some of your hurt, anger, or resentments? Whatever it may be, offer it up to the universe by repeating words like the following: "I willingly give all of this pain, all of this trauma, all of this stress back to the universe to dissolve and transform," and again repeat out loud whatever you're giving up with your symbolic offering. Maybe your next item is one of the foods you've been addicted to, and your statement of release sounds like "I am willing now to stop being a victim to this food. I now take back all the power I once gave to this chocolate cake." If you are throwing a pair of shoes away, even though you might put them in the bag of your past, at the end of the ceremony you might want to put them in another bag to give away to someone who can actually wear them. If indeed they are getting thrown out, talk about all the ways the shoes have been too small, too tight, too crippling. Let the shoes be symbolic of the self you're leaving behind. (And if you don't have a pair, draw them.)

- Remember to use your breath throughout the ceremony, knowing that it's the great tool you have to help you digest and release the pain of the past and to help you connect to the divine resource that has always got your back and is steadfastly there to guide you.

- If you're not burning your items, take some salt and sprinkle it all over that bag, affirming that its contents are now washed off of you—that you're breaking the cords of the past and surrendering it to God. Bless it all, asking that you retain the soul gifts that these hurts, heartaches, failures, and losses were meant to give you. But now the past—*your past*—belongs in God's hands. Tie the bag up, wrap a bow on it if you'd like, and take it out to the garbage container. It's important that you take it out of your house or the physical space in which you live. If you have a public dumpster somewhere and you can manage to do it, I suggest you put your past in the car and take it for one last drive. You can put on your favorite music and sing your way to the dump, releasing your past with joy. If you're feeling some sadness and heartache, that's OK, too. Giving up shoes that are too small but deeply familiar can bring up feelings of loss as well. So tenderly bless whatever is there.

- When you come back from delivering your past to the trash can, it is very, very important that you get in a bath or a shower. If you can take a bath, infuse it with one cup of Epsom salts and two cups of milk. Eat some apples and honey, praying for a sweet new life. As you soak in your bath or stand under the shower, thank God over and over and over again. And thank yourself for the past you have lived and for the courage it takes to enter into and embrace the present moment.

Congratulations! You have arrived at a new day. Do not go to bed without acknowledging yourself and the powers that be for the courage it has taken to remove your old shoes and feel the living presence beneath your bare feet. Make sure that you thank yourself a thousand times. Send love to every cell of your being, and tell yourself that it's now safe to move forward into the arms of God.

SOUL FOOD
I am liberated from my past . . .
a fantastic future awaits.

MORNING PRACTICE:
IGNITING YOUR FREEDOM FLAME

- What is the condition of your freedom flame right now?

- On a scale of one to ten, where would you rate it? Where would you like it to be at the end of the day?

- What is your intention for the day? What intention can you create to strengthen and fuel your freedom flame?

- What is the primary feeling you want to generate from your intention?

- What will you need to do to ensure that your intention becomes a reality?

- What will you have to give up—what thought, belief, or behavior—to ensure that you fulfill your intention for today?

- What healing mantra—what sentence or phrase—can you repeat to yourself throughout the day to soothe your soul and manifest your intention?

- How many times throughout the day do you need to hear this?

The Power of Responsibility

Now that you have been liberated from the past and taken off the tight shoes you've worn for so many years, it is imperative that you begin today with a new commitment to love, honor, protect, and respect the vulnerable, beautiful you that you are. It is your job to care for this sacred being who now stands before you and recognize that it needs you to be an emotional adult who is here for the sole purpose of tending to its heart's and soul's desires. To care for this new you at the highest level, the agent of change that you must invoke today is the power of *responsibility*.

This is not the responsibility of yesterday. It is not a burden, a problem, or an afterthought. This is the sacred responsibility of choosing to hold and nourish a piece of God. This is the purpose that you long to fulfill—to cherish and nurture this holy soul that exists within you. When you are invoking the agent of change called responsibility for your life, for your happiness, and for your soul's expression, you are infused with the power of the most high. You are infused with a mission powerful enough to change the way you think, the way you act, and the way you move in the world. You are present to the fact that nobody is coming to save you, nobody is coming to care for you, nobody can shepherd this soul into the life it was meant to live but you. You are the mother, the father, the sister, the brother, the teacher, and the guide for the soul that has been placed in your trust. You are the lover, the caregiver, and the protector who, in partnership with the Divine, can and will deliver this soul of yours to its greatest destiny. Responsibility calls on you to be single-focused, to know that the only business that is yours is discerning what is God's business. God's business is the deliverance of the soul's highest expression.

Take a deep breath, and say out loud, "There is no one who can do this better than me. I was born to manifest the glory of God within me. And the only way to do this is to take my soul by the hand, bow to its every need, and humbly take the steps to lead me to the promised land."

CLEANSING RITUALS

- Today, examine the following question: "If I were being 100 percent responsible for the deliverance of my soul's expression, what would I do today? What boundaries would I set? What choices would I make? What would I let go of? Whom would I let go of? What would I open up to? What would I feed this soul? How would I clothe it? How would I care for it?" If you were 100 percent responsible for this piece of God, what would you do? And, more important, what would you not do? Make a list.

- As the emotional adult that you are today, write a letter to your soul telling it what a great honor it is to be the keeper of its flame, to be its partner and humble servant in ensuring that God's light gets expressed through its divine mission.

SOUL FOOD
I am a responsible adult who thrives in the world.

MORNING PRACTICE:
IGNITING YOUR RESPONSIBILITY FLAME

- What is the condition of your responsibility flame right now?

- On a scale of one to ten, where would you rate it? Where would you like it to be at the end of the day?

- What is your intention for the day? What intention can you create to strengthen and fuel your responsibility flame?

- What is the primary feeling you want to generate from your intention?

- What will you need to do to ensure that your intention becomes a reality?

- What will you have to give up—what thought, belief, or behavior—to ensure that you fulfill your intention for today?

- What healing mantra—what sentence or phrase—can you repeat to yourself throughout the day to soothe your soul and manifest your intention?

- How many times throughout the day do you need to hear this?

The Power of
Humility

Now that you have taken full responsibility for the soul that you carry, it is imperative that you get all the support you need. To do this, you will have to stop trying to manage the thoughts, beliefs, and actions that arise from your mind and ask instead to be guided by a source greater than yourself. You will need to ask for assistance and for courage. By asking God, "Please do for me what I cannot do for myself," you commit fully to living the humble life of a spiritual servant. Right now, here on this planet, at this momentous time in history, you must ask the Divine to deliver you to your highest possible expression and to continually lift you out of the bondage of self so that you may be able to serve all those who might be healed or inspired by your presence and gifts. You must ask for this depth of guidance so that you continually return to the realm of consciousness, where you understand and know that you are only an instrument of the Divine, here to help the entire human race evolve into its next greatest expression. It is in this spirit of pure service and vulnerable humility that you are guided to hear the voice of your soul.

When you invoke *humility*, your next agent of change, you are in touch with this holy state and its divine resonance. You are blessed with a deep connection to God that will allow you to know your true worth and understand why you are here. This is a state of consciousness worth working toward every day for the rest of your life. Humility changes you at your core and helps you to transcend the habitual responses of your lower self, to see how deeply you matter, and to know what a vital role your soul plays in the uplifting of the world.

Your mission today is to turn over your life and your will to the care of something greater than yourself. It is to consciously choose, each minute of the day, to look outside your ego's will in order to see the greater will that wants to be done. Today is the day to clean out the arrogance, stubbornness, and fear that prevent you from living in the blessed state of humility. As you reflect upon each aspect of your life, begin to notice where you are led by arrogance; notice the places where you believe you can—or must—do it on your own. Allow yourself to see the places where you are too attached to what you want, and then ask to be led to a higher perspective. Open up to the possibility that you might actually need some assistance, and imagine yourself becoming open enough to receive it.

CLEANSING RITUALS

- Allow yourself to see those areas of your life in which you have been trying—unsuccessfully—to do things entirely on your own. Where have you been too arrogant or embarrassed to ask for help?

- In your journal, write down the worst possible thing that could happen if you allowed God to support you and your soul in daily life.

- For a few minutes each hour, close your eyes and repeat this powerful prayer from the third step of Alcoholics Anonymous. It is by far the most powerful prayer I have ever used, and it has delivered me to where I am today:

> God, I offer myself to thee, to build with me and to do with me as thou wilt. Relieve me of the bondage of self, that I may better do thy will. Take away my difficulties, that victory over them may bear witness to those I would help of thy power, thy love, and thy way of life. May I do thy will always.

SOUL FOOD
God can do for me what I cannot do for myself.

MORNING PRACTICE:
IGNITING YOUR HUMILITY FLAME

- What is the condition of your humility flame right now?

- On a scale of one to ten, where would you rate it? Where would you like it to be at the end of the day?

- What is your intention for the day? What intention can you create to strengthen and fuel your humility flame?

- What is the primary feeling you want to generate from your intention?

- What will you need to do to ensure that your intention becomes a reality?

- What will you have to give up—what thought, belief, or behavior—to ensure that you fulfill your intention for today?

- What healing mantra—what sentence or phrase—can you repeat to yourself throughout the day to soothe your soul and manifest your intention?

- How many times throughout the day do you need to hear this?

The Power of Acceptance

To live powerfully in the present, you must be able to accept life as it is today. If your shell has fallen away and you have begun to venture out beyond the familiar haunts of the past, you might feel a little bit off balance. So today is a day when you will find new footings and set the solid foundation for the self that you are in this moment. Today is the day when you can begin to stand more firmly and consciously in the world, knowing that you don't have to do it alone and that you are in the beginning stages of a miraculous, joy-filled future.

To stabilize your emotions and set your feet firmly in the present, you must invoke the agent of change called *acceptance*. You must accept all that you are, all that you've been, and all that you will be in the future. You must accept that while you are always free to make choices based on your ego's will, you—the grand you, the soul-inspired you—have chosen to live for divine will. Your foundation is rooted in faith rather than fear, in hope rather than resignation, and in joy rather than anger and regret. You have accepted the calling of your own soul, and this exhilarating feeling will now be the reference point from which all of your choices will be made.

To plant yourself firmly on the path of your soul's destiny, the first fact you must accept is that your past is your past and it will never be anything different. There is nothing you can do to change it. The second fact that you must accept is that shit happens—stuff happens in your world that will affect your life, and, again, there is nothing that you can do about it. Accepting these truths is a part of becoming an emotionally responsible adult and a humble servant of the divine.

You have to accept that life is filled with ambiguities, contrasts, and paradoxes, and that there will always be challenges for you to overcome. You have to accept that every challenge is really an opportunity that is meant to help you to grow, to evolve, to open up, and to reclaim wisdom from the guides beyond. You have to accept that your only job is to be the keeper of your own flame, and that in building the power and the magnificence of your own internal fire, you will be graced with the ability to ignite and inspire hundreds of other flames in the world. You have to accept that there are things you can do each day to ground yourself, to care for yourself, to expand your awareness, and to forge ahead toward your holy future.

To invoke the agent of change called acceptance, today is the day you will live the Serenity Prayer.

CLEANSING RITUALS

- As you reflect on the first line of the Serenity Prayer— "God, grant me the serenity to accept the things I cannot change"—look at your life and make a list of anything that you don't accept about your current circumstances. Then, ask yourself whether you are willing to accept that you cannot change those things.

- Reflect now on the second line of this timeless prayer: "Courage to change the things I can." Looking around at your life again, make a list of the things you can change.

- Finally, allow yourself to see what you will need to accept, embrace, release, or act on in order to make the changes you can make.

SOUL FOOD
Today I accept all the things that I cannot change.

MORNING PRACTICE:
IGNITING YOUR ACCEPTANCE FLAME

- What is the condition of your acceptance flame right now?

- On a scale of one to ten, where would you rate it? Where would you like it to be at the end of the day?

- What is your intention for the day? What intention can you create to strengthen and fuel your acceptance flame?

- What is the primary feeling you want to generate from your intention?

- What will you need to do to ensure that your intention becomes a reality?

- What will you have to give up—what thought, belief, or behavior—to ensure that you fulfill your intention for today?

- What healing mantra—what sentence or phrase—can you repeat to yourself throughout the day to soothe your soul and manifest your intention?

- How many times throughout the day do you need to hear this?

The Power of Risk

The comfort of the self that you know, even if you haven't loved it, always comes with a false sense of security that you will be tempted to hold on to. Like sleeping in your own bed and wearing your same old clothes, it brings some sort of inner security that a part of you wants to cling to. But the problem is that if you continue to stick with the same familiar habits and make the same choices each day, whether it is to turn on the television when you get home, check your e-mail at lunch, or eat the same seven meals for dinner each week, you will become stale and robotic, refusing to have your life show up any differently than it did yesterday, boring yourself and starving your soul. Your soul is infinitely creative. It is alive and expansive in nature. It is curious and playful, changing with the tides of time. So if you do not allow it to have full expression, it will curl up in a fetal position until you are ready to acknowledge the gifts that it holds and the value that it brings. This means you must invoke the agent of change called *risk,* which ensures that things will not be the same tomorrow as they are today. All real change *requires* risk. You must take risks every day of your life. You must get up each morning and ask not, "What can I do that is the same today?" but in fact the complete opposite: *What can I do that is different?*

I discovered the power of risk when I suddenly realized that I was so much happier when I was on the road in a strange town, eating at different restaurants, tasting new foods, and meeting new people. At first I was resistant to traveling because I wasn't as comfortable as when I was home with my family and my things. But one day, when I was visiting a small town in a state that I don't even like, I found myself laughing so hard, having a spontaneous and unexpected thrill eating a bowl of strange noodles topped with slimy little fish. In that moment, my whole being seemed to come alive. I realized that day that my *soul* was having fun. Even if it wasn't entirely fun for me to step beyond the confines of my life at home, it was fun for my soul. My soul woke up as I did something outside the norm. When I took risks to move beyond the borders of the self that I knew, I felt healthier, happier, and more fulfilled. And it quickly became apparent that I didn't have to be on the road in order to experience this. I could grow right inside my own hometown. I could make plans with people I didn't know, take ballroom-dance classes at a studio that I'd never entered, and wear something other than my old comfortable sweats when I walked out the door in the morning. And it's encouraging to know that change doesn't have to take a long time. After just a few short days of taking risks, I felt more alive than I had in years.

Today is the day to break free from the prison of the person you know yourself to be and step into a self you have yet to know. Will it be comfortable? No, but do it anyway. Growth is usually uncomfortable. If you're looking for comfort, you will more than likely feel tired and old earlier than you want, and the misery of your caged soul will always be looming nearby. So do it with joy, or at least with curiosity, because all living things must grow or they die—even you.

CLEANSING RITUALS

- Surprise yourself. If you typically keep your mouth shut when you are in groups of people, say just one thing, even if it's "I can't keep my mouth shut any longer." If you brush your teeth with your left hand, try doing it with your right. And if you tend to make your child wrong for something that they do, try making them right or coming at it with a new approach.

- In your journal, write down the answers to the following questions, and then take action. If you are not ready to risk big every day, go over the top every other day.

  What kinds of foods could I try that I'm not familiar with or that I said I would never eat?

What newspaper or books could I read that would be outside my usual choices?

What behaviors could I consider trying today that would be unlikely for me?

What new kind of entertainment can I explore this week?

What new nighttime ritual can I do tonight before bed?

- Ask for support in living out there on your evolutionary edge. If you find it difficult to ask for support, take a deep breath and ask for it anyway. The worst that will happen is that the other person will say no and you will grow.

SOUL FOOD
Change is the magical elixir of my soul.

MORNING PRACTICE:
IGNITING YOUR FEARLESS FLAME

- What is the condition of your fearless flame right now?

- On a scale of one to ten, where would you rate it? Where would you like it to be at the end of the day?

- What is your intention for the day? What intention can you create to strengthen and fuel your fearless flame?

- What is the primary feeling you want to generate from your intention?

- What will you need to do to ensure that your intention becomes a reality?

- What will you have to give up—what thought, belief, or behavior—to ensure that you fulfill your intention for today?

- What healing mantra—what sentence or phrase—can you repeat to yourself throughout the day to soothe your soul and manifest your intention?

- How many times throughout the day do you need to hear this?

The Power of the Present

What does being present really mean? It means being here, completely here, right this moment. It means that this is all there is. There is no tomorrow or even a yesterday or a later today. *Now* is all that exists. Harnessing the power of the present means having your full awareness on the task at hand and merging with the moment. That is why the *present* is our next agent of change. It's realizing that this instant in time is unlike any you've experienced before or will experience again. The now is here, and that's all there is.

As you are reading the words on this page, allow the experience of this moment in time to penetrate your entire consciousness. Be the word, the sentence, the printed page. Give 100 percent of your awareness to every word without distracting yourself with thoughts of the future or the past, and you will have the experience of being present. When you master the art of being fully awake to this moment, you bestow a precious gift on your soul—the experience of love. Being present is the art of the soul. Your mind is at rest because there is nowhere else to go and nothing else to do. There is no past to haunt you or pull you backward. And there is no future to wish for or fantasies to maintain. Being present is truly the demonstration of "this is as good as it gets," because nothing is real except this very moment. And now that *that* moment is gone, there is only *this* moment. Time passes, but you remain in the eternal state of now . . . the state of love.

When you become present to these words and let go of wrestling with time and resisting what *is*, you will feel a level of peace, relaxation, love, and contentment that can be accessed only in this moment. This is why it is called the precious present—because when you are in it, it is the greatest gift you will ever give yourself.

Being present means being completely aware of all that is. It means you're not in denial, you're not pretending, and you're not avoiding. When you are grounded in the present—feeling your feelings, listening to your body, tasting your food, and expressing your ideas—you do not build up toxicity. You digest your experience as you go. If you just found out, for example, that a friend of yours got hurt or that you've lost a family member, you will feel sad. But if you allow your feelings to move through you and be digested, you'll discover that you don't have to drag the feelings of that moment into the next moment.

While your past can inform you and your future can inspire you, the moment of choice exists in the here and now. By relinquishing your obsession with the past and your fantasies about the future, you can tap into the power of the present, and feel the force of love that resides inside of you.

CLEANSING RITUALS

- As you go about your life today, imagine that the present moment is all that exists. There is no past to overcome and no future to race toward. Ask yourself if what you're doing, thinking, feeling, and experiencing in this moment is bringing you joy and fulfillment. If it is, continue doing what you're doing. If it's not, make a different choice.

- Start a present-moment awareness practice today. For five minutes each hour, practice getting present. You could:

  Go outside into nature and become aware of your surroundings. Get present to the earth, to the sand, to a tree, to a flower.

  Lightly run your hands over your body to get present to your own skin, and then tune in to the sounds around you—a plane flying overhead, a dog barking, a bird tweeting.

When you're on the phone with a friend, listen to them as though you've never heard such beauty and inspiration. Listen to the sound and quality of their voice. Listen to their words, even if a complaint, with awe and fascination. Feel your body as you're listening. Tune in to all the sensations. Allow your awareness to take in the taste in your mouth, the thought in your mind, the motion in your body, just as they are.

- Take a shower and become present to all that is going on in and around your body. Notice your skin, your heartbeat, your breath, and the feel of the water traveling from your head to your toes.

- Write out a letter to yourself today. If you were completely present to the sacred vessel and vehicle of your body, how would you care for it? What would you want to say to it? What love and gratitude would you want to express?

SOUL FOOD
This precious moment is all that there is.

MORNING PRACTICE:
IGNITING YOUR LOVE FLAME

- What is the condition of your love flame right now?

- On a scale of one to ten, where would you rate it? Where would you like it to be at the end of the day?

- What is your intention for the day? What intention can you create to strengthen and fuel your love flame?

- What is the primary feeling you want to generate from your intention?

- What will you need to do to ensure that your intention becomes a reality?

- What will you have to give up—what thought, belief, or behavior—to ensure that you fulfill your intention for today?

- What healing mantra—what sentence or phrase—can you repeat to yourself throughout the day to soothe your soul and manifest your intention?

- How many times throughout the day do you need to hear this?

The Power of Truth

To live in the light of a new day and an unimaginable and unpredictable future, you must become fully present to a deeper truth—not a truth from your head but a truth from your heart; not a truth from your ego but a truth from the highest source. You have to be willing to be deeply honest with yourself about the shape your life is in each day. You've got to be honest about the good, the bad, and the ugly, about what works and what doesn't, so that you can live in accordance with your highest self. When you fail to tell the truth, you are kept bound to the past in ways that devastate your soul. The depth of your truth will, in fact, dictate where you can go, what you can have, what you can experience, what you can enjoy, and what you are asked to contribute by the higher realms. This agent of change—the *truth*—asks for total commitment. It requires that you tell the whole truth and nothing but the truth.

As you step into your limitless self, you will be confronted each day with old habits and patterns that are not necessarily based in truth. These old ways of being show up because you have repeated many of them thousands of times, so to think they won't try to sneak back into the comfort zone of your psyche would be a mistake. It takes months, often years, to stabilize new levels of consciousness and to seal the doors to the past so firmly that these old thought patterns can't come marching in whenever they like. Often they show up when you are busy, moving a bit too fast, and have your defenses down. Or they appear when you are feeling stressed because you took back the reins of your life. The old will try to reenter and be adopted by the self that you are today. Don't be tricked into believing that, once you have a day when you feel more alive and connected to your soul and to God's brilliance, you're free forever. Consciousness cannot be bought and paid for. It cannot be caged. It is an infinite pool that is vast and ever-changing, one that asks you to commit to living within a daily practice of truth. So in order to let the radiant light of your soul shine onto your daily existence, truth insists that you take a fiercely honest daily inventory of your life.

I remember a time when I thought I was living in truth. My light seemed to be shining brightly, but I kept bumping up against a wall with my physical health. I couldn't seem to get a handle on how to stay well, vital, and strong. I knew that when God is present, the truth is present, and that when spirit is present, there is a lack of dis-ease. So I invoked this agent of change by asking myself, "Where is the lie? Where is my self-deceit?" As I wrote in my journal, I was shocked to uncover this truth: I was spending more time looking good than feeling good. I was spending more time caring for others than taking care of myself. I was spending too much time looking at what wasn't working and not enough time blessing what was working perfectly. In a moment, activating this agent of change allowed me to shift from feeling like a victim to standing in the powerful truth of my inner wisdom. In seeing the truth, I shifted from the anxiety of my ego-driven perspective to the soul-centered peace of my higher self.

So why don't we tell the truth? Why do we continually get caught in the web of our ego's lies and our addictive behaviors? I assert that the answer is laziness. Laziness has us fall prey to the quick-fix mentality of the ego and ease God out of the picture. Laziness has us slide back into the ego's losing formula— "I can do it alone. I don't need any help or support"—which sparks the deceit and fuels other lies.

God is truth. Truth is the presence of the greatest expression of your soul. Anything else is, at best, a partial lie. So today, to invoke this agent of change called the truth, you must break all the agreements you have with others and with your lower self. You must admit to the hidden contracts you've adhered to in the past and open up to the sacred contracts your soul is destined to fulfill. Often you don't tell the truth, and don't even know you're *not* telling the truth, because you have agreements with other people that cause you to sell your soul rather than honor the light within. Today you must confront the lies that hold power over your destiny.

CLEANSING RITUALS

- Take an inventory of those places where you are still living inside a lie (even if it's a small one). Where are you still denying an addictive behavior? Where are you living a smaller expression of your soul's truth?

- Make a list of all the excuses, rationalizations, justifications, and stories you are telling yourself about why you have not been able to create and change this area of your life.

- Now, imagine that in each area you've identified, you made an agreement in the past that has kept this pattern in place. For example, if you are still struggling with your finances and haven't been able to move forward in manifesting your desired result, imagine that you are just fulfilling an old internal agreement that you signed in the past. If this were true, what would this agreement say? "I promise to never be more successful than my mother [or father]"? Or "I promise to always maintain the lie that money is the root of all evil"? Just close your eyes and ask yourself, "What agreements am I holding on to that are keeping me stuck in the past and creating the same results in the present?"

• Take your time, and when you find the agreements that are still negatively directing your life, write them down on a piece of paper, write "Null and Void" at the top, and then sign your name to it. Then write out new agreements that would ensure your success. If you need help with this, just close your eyes and ask your higher self to make you aware of the new agreements that would be an expression of a soul living in accordance with God's will.

• After you have written down both sets of agreements and have placed them in front of you, choose which agreements you will live by. That's right: decide which agreements are divine agreements for your soul. Then close your eyes, breathe in deeply, and tell yourself in the presence of spirit that you have powerfully chosen your future. Take the other list of agreements and tear it up into a hundred pieces, until there is nothing more to tear. When those tired old agreements have been transformed into nothing more than little shreds of paper, joyfully gather them up, take them outside, and throw them in the garbage where they belong. Now is the time to smile, breathe deeply, and send yourself some extra loving.

- To seal in the power of truth that is evident in your new, life-affirming agreements, read them over every night for one month.

SOUL FOOD
The truth will set me free.

MORNING PRACTICE: IGNITING YOUR INTEGRITY FLAME

- What is the condition of your integrity flame right now?

- On a scale of one to ten, where would you rate it? Where would you like it to be at the end of the day?

- What is your intention for the day? What intention can you create to strengthen and fuel your integrity flame?

- What is the primary feeling you want to generate from your intention?

- What will you need to do to ensure that your intention becomes a reality?

- What will you have to give up—what thought, belief, or behavior—to ensure that you fulfill your intention for today?

- What healing mantra—what sentence or phrase—can you repeat to yourself throughout the day to soothe your soul and manifest your intention?

- How many times throughout the day do you need to hear this?

The Future

As you stand at the doorway of your third week of the Consciousness Cleanse, can you feel the momentum building within you? This is the holy momentum that can support you not only in the seven days to come, but for the rest of your life. It is the soul's force that can propel you to continue breaking through the illusion of separateness and all of the confusion and senseless struggling that that misconception brings. As you continue the work of acknowledging and claiming the gifts of your past and standing in the power of your present, you are freeing up enormous reserves of creative energy. And I use the word *reserves* intentionally, in order to point out that for a lifetime you've been stockpiling countless dreams, desires, and future visions in your divine savings account and it's time now to make the transfer and let yourself have what is rightfully—and soulfully—yours. Taking your power back from the ghosts of the past and waking up to how many blessings already exist for you in the present is the sacred preparation for a future of profound fulfillment and deep joy.

Over the past fourteen days, you've tended to your internal garden with great concentration and focus, pulling up the weeds of limiting beliefs and stories and fertilizing the soil of your consciousness so that new life can emerge. Now you are ready to *reseed* your sacred garden—to deliberately and purposefully encode your consciousness with fresh, high-vibration thoughts, beliefs, feelings, and images. And I can tell you with conviction that over the next seven days you can lay the groundwork for a garden that will continue to bear fruit for all of the days of your life.

Claiming the shimmering light within our internal darkness is ultimately for this very purpose: to encode our lives with divine consciousness . . . to align our lives with God. When we finally understand that our job is to bring the holy medicines of compassion, forgiveness, and love to our wounded hearts, we find ourselves standing in this fertile, wide-open place, where we are ready to imbue our consciousness with new thought forms and soul-filled possibilities. Having purified our energetic signals and removed the toxic residue that was blocking our communication network, we naturally send out pure, high-resonance thoughts and feelings to everyone and everything around us. Our desires and dreams, now unobstructed by emotional toxicity, are communicated secretly, invisibly, directly, and immediately into the mind of God.

Can you sense the immense power of having the communication channels with your divine resource continuously open and clear? Imagine having daily access to your own inspiration hotline and the future possibilities that arise from that. And what is the inherent potential of having an extraordinary future in front of you? The future can seem very mysterious and intangible until you recognize it as one of God's greatest tools for beckoning you toward your most magnificent self. It is as if the Divine is asking you, "Who do you want to be in the future? Good! Be that now." Or "What do you want to experience, create, and contribute in the future? Good! Begin it now." By giving up wanting to have it or be it *later*, you begin to live it and be it *now*. That is the magic of the future. It asks you to step right now into the shoes of the one you are becoming. As Emmet Fox says, "[Y]our true place is calling, calling, and because you really are a Spark of the Divine, you will never be content until you answer."

I was never aware of the importance of answering the call as poignantly and acutely as I was when my son, Beau, began preparations for his bar mitzvah. Since the time he was very little I had been looking for a rabbi who would really teach him, in his soul, what it is to be Jewish—a strong guide who would help to prepare him spiritually for the transition from boyhood to manhood. I never really connected with my own

Judaism, but for some reason I was called to make sure Beau had a deeply spiritual and meaningful experience.

I remember wondering, when I was a little girl, what I was missing when it came to God, and saying to myself, "I don't get it. Something is wrong here." I remember my mother dressing me up and putting on my nice black patent-leather Mary Janes. My parents would pile my sister, my brother, and me in the car and drive us to our neighborhood synagogue. I remember that, as we began the walk into the sanctuary, what seemed liked hordes of people greeted my parents, wishing them the appropriate holiday sentiment, like *Shabbat shalom*, *L'shanah tovah*, or my least-favorite-sounding greeting of all, *Gut Yontiff* (GUT YAHN-tiff; "gut" rhymes with *put*). Inevitably, the grown-ups would look over at me and my siblings and make comments about how big we were getting or how cute we all were. And although the atmosphere was almost always friendly and jovial, I never understood what was really going on. I'm not sure how it was for my brother and sister, but I was clueless. I had no idea why we were there or what the purpose of it all was. And I certainly didn't know the English translation of the words that everyone was murmuring. I only knew that this was a place where we would read from musty old books that seemed to be put together backward (Jewish prayer books are read from right to left). We would all sing and pray, *daven* as it's called, and we would always wish each other well. It felt like a torture chamber—a place where most of us kids were miserable, anxiously waiting to be let out of the confines of the four walls of the temple so that we could run around freely on the playground outside.

In my own naive way, I understood three basic things: (1) we were born Jewish; (2) we were the chosen people; and (3) we occasionally had overly long meals where we were mandated to eat foods that I hated like gefilte fish and chopped liver. But looking back, I had far more questions than I had answers, and I could see that this was always my biggest challenge: understanding why—why we were here and what the point was. I had an inner ache to *know*. I remember asking my father, "Why do some of my friends get to make the sign of the cross when they pray? Why do they worship a Jewish man that most Jews don't even acknowledge?"

And those hours spent at the synagogue brought forth the deeper questions, like what was really supposed to be going on in shul (synagogue). With all my heart I wanted to know why this weekly ritual was so important and how it was supposed to serve me in becoming a better little girl. I wondered, Who is this God that we are here to worship, and why don't I feel any connection to Him? Where is He anyway, and why can't I see Him? And then my deeper, silent questions: If there really is an almighty God, why are there people without homes? Why do some people go without food and water, mothers and fathers? Why are people fighting and dying every day? Why do people have to suffer even when they are good people who go to shul?

From my early childhood to my teenage years, I quietly and privately struggled to understand it all and to find answers to my questions. In my disconnection from the true meaning behind the religious rituals and all the talk of God, I felt a great emptiness. Looking back, I can see that the tender years of my youth were spent painfully trying to fill the deep hole in my heart and the emptiness in my soul. When I was later blessed to become a mother myself, I knew from the start that I didn't want Beau to experience the same spiritual desolation I had grown up with. It was then, in my late thirties, that I made the decision to find a guide who would help Beau to understand the spiritual significance of the future that was calling him. Twelve years later—and one year before Beau's bar mitzvah—we found him.

One day my friend Keith, who knew I had been looking for a special teacher for Beau, told me about "the smiling Rabbi." He said, "Don't ask too many questions, just go meet him!" So I picked up the phone and made an appointment with Rabbi Baruch Ezagui. When Beau and I finally met him, Beau had a smile on his face that I had rarely seen: he was completely lit up. And I knew in those first three minutes that this was going to be Beau's rabbi. This was a man whose love of the Divine was uncontainable and unquenchable, and his faith in the significance of each and every soul on earth was unwavering. It was clear that he would be the religious and spiritual mentor who would help to instill in my precious son not only a faith in the future of our world but also a sense of the importance of his part in its unfolding.

In one of the first of many unforgettable conversations, the rabbi talked to Beau about the meaning of the word *mitzvah*, sharing with him that more than simply being a good deed, a mitz-vah is an *opportunity* to connect with God, to connect with other people, and to reach and stretch ourselves to become more than who we think we can be. To give Beau an idea about his special place in this big, wide world, and the importance he would play in the future, the rabbi talked about the beautiful music that his soul was here to make—the song that was unique to his soul. To illustrate the point, he had Beau imagine that he was in a concert hall listening to a symphony orchestra. He wanted him to imagine a classical music concert, and the multiplicity of events that must take place in order for an event of this magnitude to occur. Looking at the whole picture—the vast concert hall and the enormous amount of work that goes on behind the scenes—is truly mind-boggling. He suggested that every concert is a production that takes years to put together, from the publicist to the people who sell the tickets; from the production crew to the guy who parks the cars; from the people who wrote the music to the ushers who fill the seats.

There might be a hundred different people in the orchestra, the rabbi explained. And if you look to the side, you'll see someone holding a small, humble triangle. And with one small stick, that person hits the triangle for just one second of the entire concert. But unless this note had sounded, the concert would not have been the same. The same is true of the poster boy who put up the posters, the janitor who cleaned off the seats, and the guy who hung from the rafters with the spotlight: each plays a humble yet irreplaceable role.

The rabbi shared this story to illustrate a very important point: a mitzvah doesn't have to be earth-shattering. In the same way, the roles we play in life don't have to be earth-shattering. But as in the orchestra world, every little detail is what makes the music beautiful and creates the environment in which we can enjoy it. Can you imagine going to a concert hall that was filled with garbage, or one where half the lights were out so you couldn't see who was on the stage? Every detail combined makes the event a magical experience or a forgettable one.

The rabbi's lesson is that life is not about having our own fifteen minutes of fame and glory—even though many think it is. Instead, everyone's moments of fame and glory are intertwined. Greatness takes more than one. No one could experience their fifteen minutes of fame without the entire universe intimately conspiring to support that occurrence. So each person's contribution—even if seemingly small—is what makes the whole orchestra of society work. We just need to show up and be prepared, since at any moment we may be called on to contribute. Any moment may be our moment to play our piece of the music—and it's really not just one moment at all. It's a moment that will repeat itself over and over again, leading to someone else's moment.

Whenever we do something good, we need to know that it's only the beginning of the next good deed, because the person receiving the good deed is going to pass it on to a third person, and around and around it will go. We're all connected. We're all intertwined. There is really never a small moment; there is never a small deed. We will always have opportunities to be connected to the bigger picture, and we need to be ready. We always need to be prepared to show up so that we can deliver our contribution.

The next seven days of the cleanse are designed to help you hear your piece of the music. Within you there are songs of hope, contentment, gratitude, and love that can cleanse you of your heartache and hurt. For every painful or toxic situation you've been in, for every negative criticism you have listened to, for every bit of fear, doubt, or despair you've allowed into your consciousness, you can now counter that negativity by retuning to the melody of your soul's real purpose and destiny.

From day fifteen through day twenty-one, you will be bathing yourself in the light of your future. And as you continue to claim your gifts, declare your power, and stoke your internal flame, a marvelous thing will occur: deep within you will arise the knowledge that you are being called to be all of who you are. And more and more, you will have the high-vibration vantage point of seeing that your discontent, frustration, and emotional pain are your guides, pushing you forward even when you want to quit, even when you're tired, even when you can't take it anymore or when nothing makes sense. You will never be happy, or ever feel fully fulfilled, until you let that divine power merge with the personality that you are and show you an outlet for your unique contribution.

Remember, your soul's desire *is* the voice of God. You are being called even in this moment to unveil the next greatest evolution of yourself. You are always being called, but if you are not aware of this divine truth, you will miss out. You do not need to concern yourself with asking *how* you will step into your greatness, because the divine within you is always close by, whispering your next steps in your ears. As one of my favorite quotes reminds us, "God doesn't call the qualified, he qualifies the called." Take the next seven days to listen intently, and you will hear it. And then your next holy job is to *heed* it.

A PRAYER FOR THE FUTURE

Divine spirit, thank you for giving me the capacity for
wholeness
thank you for this very precious moment
a moment where I am present to all the goodness that exists
inside and outside of me
a moment that inspires thoughts of a greater future
a future where I can serve and be served
a future where I humbly and gracefully contribute my soul's
gifts to the world
I see it, I feel it, I acknowledge it right now
and so I know that it is

The Light of Realization

On day fifteen of the cleanse, I congratulate you. You have made it to the most magical part of this process. Emmet Fox taught me that the art of living is to make each moment as perfect as I can with the realization that I am an instrument and expression of the Divine herself. I learned that the only way to do this is to become a master at shifting my own consciousness. You can do this, too. All states of being, all levels of consciousness, are an option at all times. There is always a different point of view—a new place you can look from, and fresh eyes you can see through—that will lift you out of the darkness and into the glorious light of your higher self.

To take advantage of these divine perspectives, you must commit to the moment-by-moment practice of choosing

higher states of awareness. I like to imagine that states of consciousness are like Web sites on the Internet. There are literally
millions of sites out there in cyberspace. There is one that you
can mark as your home page, which comes up every time you
open your browser (and which in this case would be the state
of consciousness that you're most familiar with). There are a
few sites that you've bookmarked because you like to visit them
over and over again, and there are millions you've never seen.
Every Web site has a different look, feel, and message, all evok-
ing a different feeling. The same is true for states of consciousness. Every state of consciousness you visit by placing your
thoughts and awareness on it opens up different experiences,
emotions, opportunities, and ultimately a different view of reality. When you visit www.disappointment.com, for example,
you dip into the feelings of disappointment you have about
your life, your choices, or the disappointing behaviors of
others. Or on a day when you feel especially gloomy, you
might slip into resignation.com, where you are certain to find
evidence that you will never change and that your life has no
meaning or purpose.

But if you are willing to live a divinely inspired life, you
must now invoke this most powerful agent of change called *realization*. Making powerful, conscious choices based in the present is the quickest way to realization—to making your God-self
real; to embodying and expressing your holy light. To turn on
the light of realization, you must choose the new states of consciousness you want to visit and explore. You must commit to

visiting these new sites daily and soaking up all the good they have to offer. They must become your favorites, your home page, and your information highway for the rest of your time on earth. Any of these divine, high-vibrational states of consciousness—joy, happiness, peace of mind, contentment, gratitude, and more—are available to you right now and will remain available to you in the future. These are what you must choose if you are to live each day basking in the light. Bookmark them or type their names into your browser, and they will appear. It's your choice. Just hit Enter.

CLEANSING RITUALS

- Choose three sacred and holy frequencies that will be the foundation for your future, values that you will base your choices on, feelings that are an expression of your deepest heart. Examples include abundance, compassion, honesty, integrity, mastery, power, service, and wisdom.

- To bookmark these levels of consciousness, gather images, prayers, poems, and songs that remind you, inspire you, and evoke their vibrations within you.

- Make a list of behaviors or practices you can engage in each week that will serve as an anchor for the levels of consciousness you wish to cultivate. Choose something simple that will remind you to spend time steeping yourself in the high-resonance states that are in alignment with the future that's calling you. For example, is there an actual Web site you can visit for a few minutes each week that represents your fully realized self?

- Set yourself up for success: What can you read each morning that will set the tone for the day and remind you of your greatness? Who can you partner with to remind yourself that you are free to roam the entire spectrum of human and divine consciousness? What future can you be present to that will excite, stimulate, and leave you feeling blessed and protected? What love can you give to yourself that will leave you feeling confident and determined? Make a list of all the thoughts and words that will lift you out of your human patterns into the loving arms of divine grace.

SOUL FOOD
I am an instrument of God and I love it!

MORNING PRACTICE:
IGNITING YOUR JOYOUS FLAME

- What is the condition of your joyous flame right now?

- On a scale of one to ten, where would you rate it? Where would you like it to be at the end of the day?

- What is your intention for the day? What intention can you create to strengthen and fuel your joyous flame?

- What is the primary feeling you want to generate from your intention?

- What will you need to do to ensure that your intention becomes a reality?

- What will you have to give up—what thought, belief, or behavior—to ensure that you fulfill your intention for today?

- What healing mantra—what sentence or phrase—can you repeat to yourself throughout the day to soothe your soul and manifest your intention?

- How many times throughout the day do you need to hear this?

The Light of God's Will

God has a plan for you; I can promise you that. It's not that you're special, and it's not that you're not special. It's that your life is sacred. There is and always has been a path for your soul, and if you follow that path, it will lead you to the inner utopia that your soul longs to experience in this lifetime. You are here to manifest the glory of the Divine in a way that will serve your own soul and serve the evolution of other souls as well. What you do and how you do it matters. What you say and how you say it matters. What you choose to dedicate your time to matters, not just for you but for all those who are affected by the withholding or the deliverance of your unique gifts. You may not believe you have anything special to give, but this is just not the case. It's just the ego's voice disguising itself as a trusted friend. But you don't have to listen to it. Your gift is precious, needed, and yours to be shared and enjoyed. It is not only for the fulfillment and satisfaction of your soul but to aid all others in their evolution as well.

Your soul's mission is always to serve in the grandest way it can and to support you in growing and evolving in new ways. Divine plans lay imprinted in your inner world, and there are important lessons for you to learn and share on this journey to your most magnificent self. If you fail to see or learn the lessons, they will eventually become your limitations. Then, instead of joyfully following the voice of your highest self, you will be rerouted down a dark road filled with obstacles, limitations, and frustrating delays. So to ease on down the road, you must stay awake and aware, take direction, and follow the signs to your highest destination. The only way I know to do this is to invoke our next agent of change, called *God's will*. When you activate this change agent, your life will be forever altered. You will no longer be confused as to what path you should take, because you will be privy to the path of your own soul. You will no longer have to stay stuck, because you will just ask God to show you your next right actions, trusting that God's will for you is greater than your ego's path.

God's will can become your internal reference point from this day forward; it is your choice—God's will or your ego's will. Remember, there are no promises that can satisfy your ego's insatiable hunger for power, greed, control, or success.

There is no insurance policy big enough to calm your ego's fears that its needs will not be met. So you will have to choose: Are you going to trust the path that you've known, the path that has limited you in some way? Or are you going to roll the dice and bet all your resources on a power greater than yourself, a source that literally has the power to change everything in your life? Are you going to take a chance on a power that can open up new opportunities where there have been none, a force that will bring people out of the woodwork to support you, or will you stay stuck where you are? You have to decide. Will you commit to spending each day for the rest of your life taking direction from a power greater than your ego's limitations? Will you follow the inner and outer signs that will lead you to the next greatest evolution of your soul? Or will you hold on to the self that you know?

This is a turning point like no other. If I have any influence over your choice right now, let me encourage you to think long and hard. Go over all the ways your ego has left you high and dry, all the ways it has tricked and manipulated you, all the ways it has failed to deliver you the results you know you deserve in the areas of your life that are the most challenging for you.

Then, take control. Take your power back from your ego. Use this point as a demarcation. Raise a white flag to your higher self, and joyfully surrender yourself into the arms of God. This is a choice you'll never forget or regret.

CLEANSING RITUALS

- Look at the areas of your life where you don't have all that you desire and deserve.

- Reflect on each item on your list and ask, "Is this a desire of my ego's will, or is this God's will?"

- Now make a list of all the patterns and self-defeating behaviors in the areas where you are stuck.

- For each of the obstacles or limitations on your list, imagine new actions to take and new lessons to be learned if you were to follow God's will. Write down these new actions and any lessons your soul might still need to learn.

- Close your eyes and decide now if you will choose God's will or your ego's will.

- If you've chosen your ego's will, there is nothing to do. Business will continue as usual. If you've chosen God's will, write out a powerful statement that will remind you of your decision and inspire you moment by moment for the rest of your life. It could be as simple as "I choose God's will" or "I trust that God's will is in my highest service" or "I give myself into the arms of God."

- Now decide the number of times that you will repeat this powerful statement to yourself each day. Find five places to post reminders of your choice. You might put it as a screen saver on your computer or download a desktop wallpaper from my Web site debbieford.com/consciousnesscleanse. Put a note in your wallet, on your desk, and in your car. Remember, it is a state of consciousness that must be invoked over and over and over again.

- Make a list of the benefits that you will receive from allowing God's will to be your guide. How will it affect your life—your finances, your health, your stress level, your productivity, your relationships with others? Write out this list and make a commitment to read it for 21 days when you get up in the morning and when you go to sleep at night. It shouldn't take you more than 20 seconds. You can do it! The surprises and magic that will come into your life as a result of choosing God's will are worth any time you have to put into it.

SOUL FOOD
May I do thy will always.

MORNING PRACTICE:
IGNITING YOUR PARTNERSHIP FLAME

- What is the condition of your partnership flame right now?

- On a scale of one to ten, where would you rate it? Where would you like it to be at the end of the day?

- What is your intention for the day? What intention can you create to strengthen and fuel your partnership flame?

- What is the primary feeling you want to generate from your intention?

- What will you need to do to ensure that your intention becomes a reality?

- What will you have to give up—what thought, belief, or behavior—to ensure that you fulfill your intention for today?

- What healing mantra—what sentence or phrase—can you repeat to yourself throughout the day to soothe your soul and manifest your intention?

- How many times throughout the day do you need to hear this?

The Light of Devotion

When you are fully present to the fact that you and you alone are responsible for choosing your path and that it will never be forced on you, you will step into the light of your divine journey. When you take responsibility for the choice to live according to God's will and not your own, you are suddenly empowered to do whatever is necessary to live in the light, to choose the path of your soul, and to put your relationship with God first. When you finally muster up the courage and the strength from inside your human self to declare, "I am going to fulfill my highest potential now," you are lifted out of the confining walls of your ego's will and into the limitless grace of God's will. When your eyes are finally open and your consciousness cleansed, you see that you are either committed to expressing your soul's passion or committed to the same limitations you faced yesterday. Your choices become easier, your path clearer, and your focus more defined.

When you are committed to living a life in service to the most high, the choices to be great, to serve and be served, to love and be loved are apparent. Your spiritual, emotional, and physical flame is your number-one priority. You are keenly aware that the only way to get yourself to where you and God want you to go is to keep yourself fully bathed in the light. You know that your one and only job is to nurture and nourish yourself and the divine and holy resource within and to know that there is no one on this earth more important than you. Your life and your light are the only things that matter right now.

To stay in this constant state of inspiration and to presence the profound resource that resides within, you must invoke the agent of change called *devotion*. Devotion begins at home, inside your own awareness. Devotion is the agent of change that invites you to return to your eternal palace and get rejuvenated every day. Devotion has you shift your priorities from an outer-driven life to an inner-inspired life. Devotion is essential for fully realizing your soul's calling. It calls on you to give up control of the outer world and take control of your inner relationship with God. It literally means *to devote yourself*—minute by minute, hour by hour, and day by day—to chipping off whatever is in the way of your golden essence, anything that keeps your light from shining brightly. Devotion requires that you enter into the realm of divine consciousness, where your single core commitment is to manifest the glory of God from the inside out. That means that you do not refer to your past in order to choose how to respond or react in any given situation but instead choose from your present commitment, your only commitment, which is to be the highest, most vibrant expression of divine light that is possible for you. That is a commitment worthy of your dedication, loyalty, . . . and devotion.

Daily devotion ensures that you will walk among the masters, sing the song of your soul, and bring love and light with you wherever you go. Maybe you are asking yourself, "How can Debbie be so certain of this?" I am certain because devotion to a power greater than yourself is the doorway out of the human mind and into the heart of God.

So enjoy.

CLEANSING RITUALS

- Make a list of what you've been devoted to that no longer serves you. For example, you may have been devoted to your past, to suffering, to pleasing others, to surviving, or to making yourself feel better through the consumption of cookies. Allow yourself to explore where your devotions currently lie.

- Write your own story of divine devotion: What would be possible for your life if you were completely devoted to making your own light shine? What new choices can you make that will reflect your commitment to expressing your divine light? What is imperative that you do each day in order to allow your golden essence to be visible to the world? What future would you have to be present to to stay devoted to your highest self and your highest expression?

SOUL FOOD
Devotion is the doorway into my soul.

MORNING PRACTICE:
IGNITING YOUR INSPIRATION FLAME

- What is the condition of your inspiration flame right now?

- On a scale of one to ten, where would you rate it? Where would you like it to be at the end of the day?

- What is your intention for the day? What intention can you create to strengthen and fuel your inspiration flame?

- What is the primary feeling you want to generate from your intention?

- What will you need to do to ensure that your intention becomes a reality?

- What will you have to give up—what thought, belief, or behavior—to ensure that you fulfill your intention for today?

- What healing mantra—what sentence or phrase—can you repeat to yourself throughout the day to soothe your soul and manifest your intention?

- How many times throughout the day do you need to hear this?

The Light of Transcendence

If you devote yourself to God's will, you will need to increase your feelings of worthiness in order to step into the enormity of what's possible for your life. This is an inside job that requires you to be present to the fact that you are an extension of God, a molecule of the greatest power that exists, and that you are here to deliver a divine gift to the world. You are on a soulful path, and while on that path you have a duty to step into the greatest version of yourself. You must do this so that you can experience what's possible—not only for yourself, but for every soul on this planet. If you wish to remain in the illusion that you are separate from the whole, acting on your own accord, you will more than likely sabotage any greatness that you do express. Why? Because the deep feelings of unworthiness that arise as a result of denying your divinity will cause you to act out in ways that you never intended. To live into the grandness and expansiveness of your future, you must invoke the next agent of change, called *transcendence.*

You must transcend the "I" of your individual humanity. Your human "I" will never feel worthy enough of expressing the greatness of God's gifts. But the "we" of your divine birthright—the one that is aware of its place as part of the collective whole—knows that it is your sacred obligation to shine your brightest light, not just in your moments of glory but each day. Your "I," in all its narcissistic arrogance, will think you have actually achieved something on your own, but your collective self realizes that when you attain greatness, you have done so because you have been willing to be used by a power greater than yourself—not to just serve yourself but to inspire and ignite a light inside of each soul who is touched by your gifts, contributions, and achievements. This is how you expand a genuine sense of worthiness in yourself. This is how transcendence acts as an agent of change to light up the world.

In order to amplify the transformational power of transcendence, you must avoid claiming personal credit for your gifts. You must simply bless them and thank God for using and working through you. You must be a humble servant and know that you never act alone. This is the wisdom that will serve you when you are on the top *and* when you are on the bottom. And if you wish to know in every cell of your being that you are never alone and to transcend all the noisy internal chatter that exists within your "I," all you have to do is drop inside and ask for grace, guidance, and ease—the three signs of God's will.

CLEANSING RITUALS

- Write out all the places where you are still doing it alone, where you are stuck in the "I" that chants, "I have to do it, I can't do it, I don't know how to do it." Notice how long you've been trying to do it alone.

- Now imagine that you are an extension of God, that you've transcended your "I" and have resumed your place as a part of the collective whole. How would you act in the world if you knew you were actually a "we" and that you were not alone? Who would you ask to support you, to guide you, and to mentor you? How many minutes a day would you go inside to connect and ask God how you can serve the greater whole?

- At the end of this day, look to see what signs of God's will were evident in your day. What *grace, guidance,* and *ease* did you experience today?

SOUL FOOD
Oneness lifts me up where I belong.

MORNING PRACTICE:
IGNITING YOUR GRATITUDE FLAME

- What is the condition of your gratitude flame right now?

- On a scale of one to ten, where would you rate it? Where would you like it to be at the end of the day?

- What is your intention for the day? What intention can you create to strengthen and fuel your gratitude flame?

- What is the primary feeling you want to generate from your intention?

- What will you need to do to ensure that your intention becomes a reality?

- What will you have to give up—what thought, belief, or behavior—to ensure that you fulfill your intention for today?

- What healing mantra—what sentence or phrase—can you repeat to yourself throughout the day to soothe your soul and manifest your intention?

- How many times throughout the day do you need to hear this?

The Light of Purpose

Standing in the collective heart of humanity, you begin to be pulled toward your unique contribution to the world. Uncovering your soul's purpose is not always the easiest task. Throughout your life, you've been influenced by what you have done in the past, what you have been told you can and cannot do, and what your present circumstances seem to dictate. So in order to reveal the gifts that lie beneath the surface of your heart's greatest desires, you must now invoke the next agent of change called *purpose.*

You must not look to your past or even your present to see why you are here or what your part in the future of humanity is. You must instead look beyond your years here on earth, reconnect with the Divine, and bring forth your soul's legacy into the present moment.

An entire life can be lived yet forgotten so very quickly. Even if you are blessed with family members who love you and friends who adore you, after you're gone, in a matter of years—or sometimes months—the memory of you can become just a fleeting thought in your loved one's minds. But you can satisfy your soul's mission by committing to leaving something behind on this planet that will make a difference to those who come after you. You will die in peace, knowing that you left your soul's gift. You will have given to the world a small gift that left it a little better than when you came in.

Although you may feel overwhelmed or depressed by this conversation, I think it's imperative, if you are to find and live your soul's purpose, to thoroughly examine the legacy you hope to leave behind. Imagine that your life's efforts serve as a mark of God and that the only way the Divine gets seen, heard, or expressed is through the legacy you leave behind. The yearning to make a difference is your need to express your purpose and derive meaning from your time on earth. Although at this moment you may be unaware of your longing to leave a legacy, your legacy is your birthright, your imprint, and a purpose worth getting up for each morning. Your soul has an innate desire to leave its mark, and it is calling you, unceasingly, toward its fulfillment.

In my years of coaching and training people, I have noticed that whenever I enter into this conversation, people feel the pressure to create some grand gesture somewhere in the future, a fantasy that may never get fulfilled. It becomes a to-do instead of a "Thank God," a "someday, one day" fantasy when it should be a lifelong pursuit. There is no legacy too great or too small. It's easy to point to the legacy of Martin Luther King Jr. and how he addressed racial bondage in his lifetime, but no less significant is the legacy of the janitor from Alabama who worked hard every day making sure the children had a clean and safe place to learn.

No matter where you are or what you do, no matter where you live or what talents you were born with, you have the ability to leave a legacy that will live on beyond your time. This is your birthright to claim and the hallmark of a fully realized soul. Heed the call of your soul. Your legacy is your soul's purpose and contribution. And your time to deliver it is now.

CLEANSING RITUALS

Today is the day to reflect on the enduring meaning you want your life to have in the years following your death.

- Make a list of what you want said about you five, twenty, and fifty years after you die.

- Begin to create a vision and a plan for the legacy you want to leave behind. Ask yourself the following questions to see what kind of legacy you would like to leave behind:

If my soul is yearning to leave an imprint on the world, what would I leave?

If I am the voice of God, what could I say?

If I am the hands of the Divine, what would I create, expand, or explore?

If I am the only one who can leave my unique legacy, what is important for me to do or take on?

- Allow yourself to see what you can do right now to begin fulfilling the legacy you want to leave behind. If preserving your family's history is important to you, for example, you might choose to research and create a family tree that future generations can study and learn from. You could make a video for family and friends to express your love and share the parts of your life that are most important to you. You might get inspired to finally finish a painting or a piece of poetry that has been alive within you for months or years.

- Dwell in the realization that life is very short and your legacy cannot be postponed. And now notice how your life is infused with greater intention and meaning.

SOUL FOOD
It's safe to share my gifts with the world.

MORNING PRACTICE:
IGNITING YOUR PASSION FLAME

- What is the condition of your passion flame right now?

- On a scale of one to ten, where would you rate it? Where would you like it to be at the end of the day?

- What is your intention for the day? What intention can you create to strengthen and fuel your passion flame?

- What is the primary feeling you want to generate from your intention?

- What will you need to do to ensure that your intention becomes a reality?

- What will you have to give up—what thought, belief, or behavior—to ensure that you fulfill your intention for today?

- What healing mantra—what sentence or phrase—can you repeat to yourself throughout the day to soothe your soul and manifest your intention?

- How many times throughout the day do you need to hear this?

The Light of Compassion

As you look powerfully into the future and commit to living a devotional life—one grounded in love, care, and kindness—you open yourself up to being touched by and receiving the heart of God. What does this mean? It means that the divine heart becomes your compass. You no longer look to your own hurts or judgments to determine how you feel about yourself or others, but instead you look through God's heart to influence your thoughts, feelings, and perceptions. The divine heart knows that you and I are here to learn, grow, and evolve. It is the heart of clear perspective and the only real detector of the holy truth. The divine heart *feels* the presence or absence of authenticity, honesty, and realness and can see the greater picture of your life. It is the deeper heart, the heart of the people, the collective heart that beats as one.

As an individual with limited experience of other people's realities, you can see only what you can see. Because you cannot live in every country and practice every religion—as a German, Jew, Muslim, Latino, Asian, Lebanese, Cuban, Iraqi, Dane, Christian, Hindu, and on and on—it is impossible for you to see the full picture of what every experience actually could mean for your life. Because you can't simultaneously experience what it is to be a man, woman, infant, adolescent, adult, and retiree, you cannot access the eyes and understanding of the entire collective heart. You see yourself, others, and life itself through the only filters you have access to, which are your own. Your individual human perception allows you to see things, people, and experiences only through your own wants and needs, through your likes and dislikes, which are all influenced by your history—where you were born, how you were raised, and who you decided to be and not to be. If you go into the future truly committed to accessing the highest vibrations known to man and God, and you commit to the highest expression of your soul, you must invoke today's agent of change, called *compassion*.

Compassion is the key to living outside the confines of the ego's limitations and having an expanded perception of reality. Compassion is the healing agent that will support you every day in releasing the past and stepping into the future with calm and certainty. Compassion doesn't say, "What can the world do for me?" but rather, "How can I serve the world?" Compassion is the feeling you access when looking at the world through the eyes of the divine heart. It fears nothing, because it knows it is everything. Its judgments are limited to protecting itself, for it knows that God has a bigger plan that neither you nor I can see. A compassionate heart will lift you out of the pain and suffering of your own world, because it knows that everyone is doing the best they can, given their state of consciousness and the histories they're dragging behind them. The divine heart knows that people don't decide at age three to grow up and be a wife beater, an out-of-integrity politician, an abusive mother, a bullying neighbor, or a mediocre couch potato. Compassion knows that the gravitational pull of your history is so strong that it often wins the war between the light and the dark. So when this agent of change is activated in your awareness, you are finally free to stop taking everything so personally. You're able to step out of the perspective you are so accustomed to—the myopic view of your individual self—and instead reach to the heavens and look through the heart of God. What an astonishing view . . . and what a profound relief. It is here that you will finally find the peace you are looking for. It is here that you will be free to surrender your judgments, and it is here that you will experience the liberation of your soul.

CLEANSING RITUALS

Today is the day to consciously choose a grander and greater perspective—a perspective infused with compassion. As you do the following exercise, notice that by deliberately altering the way you look at things, you also create a shift in your perception. Notice how your awareness, intuition, insight, and spiritual discernment all come more fully alive in the process.

- In your journal, write down three pivotal, life-changing events in your life. In a nutshell, what happened, when, and who else was involved?

- Now look at each of the three events through three sets of eyes:

  Your own eyes—how you see this event

  The eyes of another significant person involved in or impacted by the event

  The eyes of the divine heart—the compassionate eyes of God

- If you were to look through the most compassionate eyes, which eyes would those be, and what would you see?

- What empowering new interpretation of this experience do you see through those eyes? What do you understand now that you didn't before? What gifts can you now see and claim?

- Allow yourself to imagine that there is a divine story of your life waiting to be revealed, a story that is important and life-changing. Imagine that you're standing in the center of your divine heart and that you are able to see a spiritual meaning that evokes your compassionate heart. Write it down in all its detail and glory. Allow this new story to shift the way you see life from this day forward.

SOUL FOOD
God's eyes are my eyes.

MORNING PRACTICE:
IGNITING YOUR COMPASSION FLAME

- What is the condition of your compassion flame right now?

- On a scale of one to ten, where would you rate it? Where would you like it to be at the end of the day?

- What is your intention for the day? What intention can you create to strengthen and fuel your compassion flame?

- What is the primary feeling you want to generate from your intention?

- What will you need to do to ensure that your intention becomes a reality?

- What will you have to give up—what thought, belief, or behavior—to ensure that you fulfill your intention for today?

- What healing mantra—what sentence or phrase—can you repeat to yourself throughout the day to soothe your soul and manifest your intention?

- How many times throughout the day do you need to hear this?

The Light of Possibility

The world is waiting for you. Inspired by the depth of your courage and strength, the Divine opens its arms to you as a fully integrated being who carries the seeds of hope, health, happiness, and prosperity. Your consciousness is fertile; it is rich with the food of your soul and the healing balm that can be offered only by your own heart. It has been through the tremendous process of cleansing and letting go, opening up, and taking in. The ground is now prepared for you to continue to plant the seeds of your greatest desires as you enter back into the world, one moment at a time and invoke our last agent of change, called *possibility*.

This reentering should be done with grace, clarity, and ease—a slow opening up to the outer world once again, but this time with new awareness, allowing only what will nourish and nurture you into the field of your consciousness. There is no rush, nowhere to go, and nothing you have to do to stay in this holy process except to remember that the relationship with your inner resource and the brilliance of your internal flame are your top priorities. Now is the time to set new boundaries, to make the words "No, thank you" your friend, so when you are asked to do something that isn't in your highest interest or that doesn't fuel your flame, you have the option to just say no. In the words of one of my favorite spiritual teachers, Alice Bandy, "Every time you say yes when you mean no, you are training yourself to deny your soul's truth and to ignore your inner knowing." Can you tally all the times you didn't listen to yourself because you wanted to be nice to someone else? When you don't trust that your instincts and intuition are correct, you shut off your inner guide. You're actually forfeiting your innate GPS, which is programmed to direct you to the destination of your dreams. Your intuitive no's are saying, "Wrong direction: don't go left, it's really a right. If you take this turn, it is going to take you much longer to get where your heart longs to go." The voice from within is your own personal guide telling you, "If you take your own route, you will probably get lost for a while. You will find other destinations, but they won't be the ones that will take you to the most high." Or maybe your GPS (God's Positioning System) is trying to get your attention by manifesting itself as a tightness in your belly, because it knows you are deaf to its voice, warning you that you will have to backtrack and make a U-turn in order to get on your path again. Within you lies one of the greatest tools ever designed to ensure your soul's fulfillment. It is programmed to tell you when you are heading toward purpose and meaning, and to alert you with feelings of happiness and joy when you arrive safely at your destination. And again, it's one of those amazing lessons, because this priceless resource is free and comes already installed in the operating system of your soul. It's part of the divine package. All you have to do is choose to acknowledge that you have it and then commit to using it. You just have to turn it on, listen closely, and do what it says. If you are courageous enough to choose to use your GPS each day and follow its directions at all times, you will arrive at the doorway of your soul's destination without all the stress and suffering of a person who's driving in a new city without a map. This is your choice.

To follow the call to new, uncharted land, you must trust in the possibilities that exist. You will have to do some things that are counterintuitive and different from the way you have been living your life. You might find yourself back in school, living in a city you thought you would never live in, making amends to someone you have hurt, or cutting back on your spending. Or maybe you will find yourself setting firmer boundaries—saying no to things you don't want to do and speaking out in situations where in the past you would have withheld your voice. The opportunities and possibilities are endless. The challenges and the losses, the shifts and the changes, will be plentiful, but the goal of a soul that is satisfied, filled up, in-spired, happy, passionate, and fully alive is worth everything you will go through on your journey.

When you are feeling good about the road you traveled at the end of each day—when you have trusted in a power greater than yourself and listened to the directions of your heart rather than your head—you will have arrived back in the land of milk and honey. It is in this place that you feel nurtured and alive. It is here that you are inspired by who you are, not what you do. It is in this higher state of consciousness that you experience being "turned on" by life, along with all the twists and turns that are a natural part of the road.

This is a trip worth taking. It is worth a long, slow drive across the county. This promised land is worth any amount of discomfort you might have to go through to become a clean, clear vessel of divine love and expression. So bask. Bask in the glory of your most divine self. Bask in the wisdom that you are an infinite source of love, joy, and hope for all humankind. Bask in knowing that within you are seeds of greatness that—if con-sistently watered and cared for—will grow into a future that will leave this planet a better place than when you arrived. You hold the map to the greatest expression of your own soul. You and only you have the directions programmed into your soul to deliver a life beyond your wildest dreams—a life where you and the Divine are one; a life where you are thrilled at being who you are, doing what you are doing, and contributing the gifts that only you bring . . . a life worth praying for.

CLEANSING RITUALS

Today marks the dawning of a new day; the birth of a new era. From this point forward, you can continuously nurture, honor, and celebrate the instincts and intuition that are sparked by your soul. The rituals and action steps on this final day of the cleanse will support you in hearing the call of your soul with ever-deepening clarity.

- Joyfully make a list of all the people and things you need to say no to at this time. See which friends don't make the needle move up on your soul's joy meter. Which old relationships, old patterns, and things from the past are still hanging around like piles of stale laundry? You really do not need them any longer. Get rid of them now.

- Commit to spending ten minutes in the morning, ten minutes in the afternoon, and ten minutes in the evening going inside and checking in with your personal GPS— seeing if you made wrong turns, seeing if you're going down the wrong road, and seeing where it wants you to go next. If you discover that you are going down a dead-end street, just stop and turn around. See what you can do to get back on track. Ask yourself, "How am I feeling? Does this choice leave me feeling holy, soulful, God-centered? Or does it make me feel insecure, fearful, or uncomfortable?" Now remember, this is a trick question, because when you start doing things in a new way, you probably will feel a little insecure, fearful, and uncomfortable. But if something feels really off, you probably need to reach out and get help. Today would be the day to do it.

- Make a list of the signs your soul is trying to give you and the signals it uses to send its messages. Are there warning signs that you get? Are there feelings of spontaneous joy that are also signs? Identify as many signs as you can.

- Make a list of all the times you had an intuitive knowing but diminished its importance or fully denied it. Use this list to acknowledge that God has been your guide all along, even when you've shown up with deaf ears. Make a commitment now to forgive yourself.

- Write a story now of your soul's purpose. Don't think about it. Just finish this sentence. "My soul's purpose is..." And then know this is indeed the truth. Now close your eyes and affirm you will do whatever it is that will fulfill that future. And together we say, "And so it is."

SOUL FOOD
I am the light of the world.

MORNING PRACTICE:
IGNITING YOUR POSSIBILITY FLAME

- What is the condition of your possibility flame right now?

- On a scale of one to ten, where would you rate it? Where would you like it to be at the end of the day?

- What is your intention for the day? What intention can you create to strengthen and fuel your possibility flame?

- What is the primary feeling you want to generate from your intention?

- What will you need to do to ensure that your intention becomes a reality?

- What will you have to give up—what thought, belief, or behavior—to ensure that you fulfill your intention for today?

- What healing mantra—what sentence or phrase—can you repeat to yourself throughout the day to soothe your soul and manifest your intention?

- How many times throughout the day do you need to hear this?

Soul Power

There is just one thing we are seeking: true peace. Nothing else matters. With peace there is love. With peace there is compassion. With peace there are the sweet stillness of serenity and the thrill of both the present moment and the future that awaits. With the presence of peace, outer actions are influenced by the inner safety of a protected life, and we naturally and willingly take risks that ensure that our soul's purpose prevails.

To experience the peace of your soul you must enter a state of consciousness in which you are unattached to the past, present, or future. Here you allow life to be as it is, knowing what you have control over and what you do not. With each breath you are present to the fact that this a divine moment, a moment to shine like you have never shone before, a moment to hold the whole world in your hands with a gentle thought and a kind heart. Peace of soul is the initiation to your authentic life—not life simply as you want it to be, but as it actually is right now.

When you are truly committed to experiencing the peace of your soul, you will wake up joyfully, look to your internal guidance to get your directions for the day, and then trust the directions given to you. You won't worry about how or when or why, because you will trust that someone has your back. You will remember that the direction will come, not in your time but in divine time. You'll enthusiastically let go of your perceived ideas and joyfully open up to being directed by that world-renowned architect—the multitalented Divine herself. What a privilege it is to have the number-one coach in the world at your side.

Your divine coach is standing by on the sidelines each morning, just waiting for you to enlist her support to take you all the way to the greatest expression of yourself. So let's begin, my friends, because this is what you've been waiting for your entire life.

Don't get hooked into the excuse that you don't have the time, because just as you know that you need food to sustain you and that your vehicle can't go anywhere without gas, this, too, is a necessity, not a luxury. With your coach at your side, you will play this game of life within the boundaries of the proper rules—new rules that will support you in enjoying the game, finding pleasure in the process, and experiencing joy in the journey. The new rules will support you on the days when you are feeling off your mark, not fully in shape for the day ahead. And they will refine your ability to access the most inspired and passionate levels of consciousness you ever imagined visiting.

On the days when you wake up feeling a bit off, you will read over the new rules again, allowing your perception to be shifted by these spiritual morsels that guarantee you will end the day in a better way than you began it. They will support you in rising above the gravitational pull of the past while staying fully grounded in the present. They will remind you of all that is waiting for you by calling forth the deepest desires of your uniquely individual soul. They are the rules of the holy earth game—the one where you remember that you are a divine being living a human experience, not a human being struggling to be divine. This is the game where you remember that there is a resource within that has the power to change the most difficult situations and guide you to a new, empowering circumstance. This is the sacred sport that works best when you remember that you are directed by your deep intuitive feelings and that even though those feelings may not make sense in the moment, they will make sense in the end.

The new rules are here now to remind you of who you truly are and what you are here to do every day of your life. They are a resource, a guide—a kick in the ass, if necessary—to get you back on track.

THE NEW RULES

1. Upon waking every morning, breathe deeply and ask to be reminded of why you are here and what your deepest desire is for the day.

2. Choose the level of consciousness that you want to explore today. Then write down three choices you can make that will ensure that you access this state. Remember, you are the one with the power here.

3. Step out of the past by bringing your attention fully to the task at hand, no matter how mundane. And appreciate that you are alive today.

4. Treat your body as if it is the most precious child you have ever held. Bring tender touch, nourishing foods, and joyful movement to it today.

5. Let go and let God. Surrender your worries and concerns to a power greater than yourself. Write them down before you go to sleep, and leave them outside on your doorstep (to be discarded).

6. Accept your life as it is today. Accept all the things you cannot change. Remember, there is a new day coming tomorrow. Breathe . . .

7. Acknowledge yourself for every good task you accomplish and for every good thought you think. Acknowledge yourself all day until you are blushing from the honest recognition of your accomplishments.

8. Literally take off your old, worn-out shoes and donate them to Goodwill or to the trash where they belong. Clean out and throw away whatever is taking up space around you that you no longer want or use.

9. You're an emotional adult and are fully responsible for your life—physically, emotionally, and spiritually. Acknowledge where in your life your adolescent self is in control, and then stop acting that way by allowing your adult self to take over.

10. Admit when you are wrong. Humility is the real key to happiness. Uncover any arrogance, any stubborn insistence on being "right," that is robbing you of peace right now.

11. When you feel bored or stuck, take a risk. Do something unpredictable and out of the norm for you.

12. Release anger, resentments, and grudges as quickly as possible. Allow yourself to voice them privately and then hand them over to the divine force within.

13. Respect your body by listening to its needs and giving it the love, care, and rest that it deserves. Take one day off a week from your phone, e-mail, and texts to refuel and replenish your sacred vehicle.

14. Remember that you deserve better. Look around your life and see where you're settling for less. And then do something today to treat yourself like the god or goddess that you are.

15. Extract the wisdom from your wounds. Declare yourself educated in the area of your life where you are feeling hurt. Write out the five most important learning outcomes from this experience.

16. The truth will always set you free. Polish up your integrity by expressing yourself honestly in some area of your life where you are withholding the truth.

17. Allow divine love to fill up the container of your consciousness and wash away your human worries.

18. Remember that your brightest light can shine only when you've accepted and embraced your darkness. Give some love to a part of yourself that you have judged, rejected, or made wrong.

19. Be present to the beautiful truth that you are here on a magical journey to make peace with both your

humanity and your divinity. Feel gratitude for all of
your God-given gifts.

20. Have fun! Find pleasure in your work, with your family,
    in your day-to-day activities. Have more joy, more sex,
    and more spontaneous belly laughs.

21. The best way to get love is to give love. Give love to as
    many people today as you can. Give an extra hug to a
    friend or family member and as many compliments as
    you can to whomever crosses your path, even the
    mailman.

There is nobody else in the universe like you, no one else
with your gifts, your style, your wisdom, your exact perspective. Today you must choose to remember this truth and reclaim your power as both a human and a divine being. You
must chose to recall that you came to this earth to live a divine
plan, a plan so important, so vital, and so necessary for the
evolution of humankind.

If you choose to remember this, you will see that every major
experience of your life was trying to teach you, guide you, and
support you in understanding the significance and importance of
your life. And, even more important, each experience was designed to get you ready to deliver your soul's passion to the
world. It is you that we need. Not some plastic, made-up version
of an ego gone astray, but the *you* that you were born to be.

Be it now, and the universe will support you through heaven and hell.

Be it now for the sake of all those you love and all those who love you.

Be it now so that you may return to the land of your soul—to a deeply restful and joyous place where you and the Divine are one, a place where the greatest expression of your soul and the greatest love imaginable merge together as one—one heart, one mind, and one mission . . . all at home inside of you.

Acknowledgments

To my amazing staff and family whose love and support make it possible for me to do what I love in the world. Frankie Mazon, I couldn't live without you—you're a spiritual rock star! Julie Stroud for your dedication, brilliance, and awesome editing skills. Cliff Edwards for your wisdom and strength, Jeff Malone for always being the holder of what's possible for our lives. And Kelley Kosow, whose grounded guidance has supported us all.

To the ever-loving Debra Evans for holding the vision for this book and always sharing your heart and your beautiful words so generously and to Danielle Dorman for your genius clarity and insight. Thank you for your support.

To my sister, Arielle Ford, and brother-in law, Brian Hilliard, who work as my agents and managers. Thank you for always believing in me.

To my phenomenal HarperOne editor, Gideon Weil, whose guidance and faith inspires me to new heights. And to the committed and talented team at HarperOne, including Mark Tauber, Claudia Boutote, Suzanne Wickham, Jan Baumer, Jim Warner, Laina Adler, and Terri Leonard.

To Jeanette Reyes and Allee Brett, whose care and impeccability support me each day.

To Geeta Singh of the Talent Exchange, who guides me out into the world more and more each year with each new book.

To Marianne Wilson and her team at Global Event Source for their marketing brilliance and Web talents.

To my branding and image guru Gio Conesa of Square One Branding and his amazing partner Renée Zborowski for creating a beautiful site and vibration for the Consciousness Cleanse to live on. And to Hans Holland of StoryBoardIT who brings Gio's vision to life with impeccability and brilliance.

To Scott Cervine and Movies from the Heart for making the Golden Buddha come alive.

To Drew Heriot for brilliantly guiding me to make my work come alive. You're a genius and a fantastic strategic consultant.

To Rita Woodard, Denise Mullins, and all the selfless board members, coaches, and volunteers who serve TheCollectiveHeart.org in service to the world.

To my Earth Angels, whose wisdom and guidance have supported me in the birthing of this book: my strong and vibrant mother, Sheila Fuerst, for taking care of me and my business, Robin Johnson, Sylvia Albrecht, Suzanne Todd, Rachel Levy,

Sherry Davis, Anne Browning, Wendy Ware, Karla Dascal, and my awesome brother, Mike Ford.

To all of my devoted coaches and students who have committed their lives and time to the study of human consciousness at The Ford Institute. Your quest has propelled me into who I am. Thank you.

A special thank-you for those who continue to inspire and guide me: Deepak Chopra, Dr. David Simon, Marianne Williamson, Cheryl Richardson, Rabbi Baruch Ezagui, Yogini Henriette Rosenberg, Alice Bandy, Dr. George Pratt, Cynthia Kersey, my Mamala Dr. Edie Eger, and to the holy mother Ammachi, whose light inspires me to shine brighter each day.

And finally, to my dynamic and wise son, Beau Bressler, whose constant encouragement makes it a joy to be alive.

About the Author

Debbie Ford is a pioneering force in incorporating the study and integration of the human shadow into modern psychological and spiritual practices. Debbie, the bestselling author of seven books, is the creator of the renowned *Shadow Process Workshop* and the executive producer of *The Shadow Effect*, an emotional-gripping, visually compelling transformational documentary featuring Deepak Chopra, Marianne Williamson, and other evolutionary thinkers.

Debbie's passion and dedication to inspire men, women, and children to live fully integrated, high-functioning lives led her to create The Ford Institute, the world renowned personal and professional training organization, and The Collective Heart, a non-profit organization helping to transform education around the world. These organizations are committed to the betterment of the human experience.

Debbie Ford has a degree in psychology from John F. Kennedy University and is the recipient of the 2001 *Alumni of the Year* award for her outstanding contributions in the fields of psychology and spirituality. Additionally, she holds an honorary doctorate degree from Emerson University and an Honorary doctorate degree from the John F. Kennedy University Board of Regents.

Please visit DebbieFord.com for additional information and free tools to support you in *The 21-Day Consciousness Cleanse*.